HOW TO LIVE
WITH LOW-LEVEL
RADIATION

HOW TO LIVE WITH LOW-LEVEL RADIATION

A Nutritional Protection Plan

LEON CHAITOW
ELIZABETH KUTTER, PH.D.

Healing Arts Press
Rochester, Vermont

Healing Arts Press
One Park Street
Rochester, Vermont 05767

Library of Congress Cataloging-in-Publication Data

Chaitow, Leon.
  How to live with low-level radiation.

  Bibliography: p.
  Includes index.
  1. Radiation injuries—Prevention. 2. Radiation
injuries—Nutritional aspects. 3. Low-level radiation
I. Kutter, Elizabeth. II. Title.
RC93.C47 1987   616.9'8970654   86-30086
ISBN 0-89281-230-3 (pbk.)

Permission to reprint figures in this book has been granted by the following:
Figure 3: The periodic table. From Wiseman, F. L., 1985. *Chemistry in the Modern World*. New York, McGraw-Hill, p. 23.
Figure 4: A fission chain reaction. From Kroschwitz, J. and M. Winokur, 1985. *Chemistry: General, Organic, Biological*. New York, McGraw-Hill, p. 65.
Figure 5: Radiation exposure to the average U.S. citizen. Courtesy of the National Society of Professional Engineers, 1980. Produced for their program "Nuclear Energy: Issues and Information".
Figure 6: Cases of reported encephalitis per 1 million people in New York City. From Sternglass, E., 1986. The Implications of Chernobyl for Human Health. *International Journal of Biosocial Research* 8:7–36. Reprinted with permission of Biosocial Publications, Tacoma, WA.

Design by Hunter Graphics.

Printed and bound in the United States.

10 9 8 7 6 5 4 3 2 1

Healing Arts Press is a division of Inner Traditions International, Ltd.

Distributed to the book trade in the United States by Harper and Row Publishers, Inc.
Distributed to the book trade in Canada by Book Center, Inc., Montreal, Quebec
Distributed to the health food trade in Canada by Alive Books, Toronto and Vancouver

TABLE OF CONTENTS

ACKNOWLEDGMENTS   vii

INTRODUCTION   ix

CHAPTER ONE
RADIATION AND ITS EFFECTS   1

CHAPTER TWO
FREE RADICALS
The Consequences of Oxidation   19

CHAPTER THREE
THE FREE RADICAL SCAVENGERS AND
QUENCHERS   31

CHAPTER FOUR
MORE GENERAL PROTECTION AND
REGENERATION OF BODY TISSUES   49

CHAPTER FIVE
RADIOTHERAPY
Enhancing Its Benefits and Reducing Its Dangers   59

CHAPTER SIX
EXCLUDING THE TROJAN HORSE
Nutritional Removal of Radioactive Material
from the Body   69

CHAPTER SEVEN
THE INVISIBLE ENEMY
Sources of Radioactivity   79

APPENDIX
SUMMARY OF RADIATION PROTECTION
METHODS   89

GLOSSARY   93

BIBLIOGRAPHY   97

INDEX   103

ACKNOWLEDGMENTS

I would like to express my thanks to a number of people who have contributed substantially to the writing of this book.

I owe a debt of gratitude to my co-author, Elizabeth Kutter, Ph.D., for her substantial input to, and incisive scientific questioning of, many aspects of the book.

To Jeffrey Bland, Ph.D., for his constructive criticism and enthusiastic sharing of knowledge.

To Alex Schauss, Emanuel Cheraskin, M.D.; and Joseph Pizzorno, N.D.; for their insights and advice.

To Sarah Bomids, editor of "Here's Health," who first supported my writing on nutritional protection for radiation. Thank you.

LEON CHAITOW

I want to express my thanks to the many people who have helped and supported me in this effort:

To my colleagues Dr. Burt Guttman, Ph.D.; Dr. Neil Jacobson, Ph.D.; Dr. Robin More, N.D.; Dr. Jeff Bland, Ph.D.; Dr. Joe Pizzorno, N.D.; Dr. Laura Udell; Dr. Filip Vanzhov, N.D.; Dr. Crystal Tack, C.A., N.D.; and to my father, Tom Martin, P.E., for their encouragement through the years of my explorations in the areas of nutrition and health as well as their careful, critical reading of the manuscript and numerous excellent suggestions.

To my students, who have continually pushed me to explore and question applications of basic science to health and policy issues, solidly supporting the overcommitment that sometimes resulted, and particularly to Beth Winslow, Anna Strong, Jessy Lorion, and Sole Guarda, for their constructive suggestions on how to make difficult scientific concepts more understandable.

To my professors in radiation biology and biophysics at the University of Rochester, who whetted my interest in radiation effects, and my colleagues at the University of California, Davis, nutrition department and at the John Bastyr College of Naturopathic Medicine, who have strongly supported the excursions of a molecular biologist into the fields of nutrition and health.

To Dr. Emanuel Cheraskin and Dr. Kendar Prasad for helpful discussions and sending much useful material, as well as their pioneering work in the area of nutrition and radiation effects.

To Eung Park for his additions on the ginseng work and his assistance in various ways during completion of the manuscript.

To my secretary, Pam Udovich, for her excellent assistance and her forbearance at my use of her computer.

To our very supportive editors, Susan Davidson and Leslie Colket.

And particularly to Dr. Chaitow for the opportunity to be involved in this endeavor. It has been a real challenge to help bridge the gap between fundamental scientific knowledge, the alternative health professions, and the concerned public, particularly in an area as complex and controversial as this one. Working with him has been a pure delight. I express my strong thanks.

BETTY KUTTER

INTRODUCTION

Since the Chernobyl disaster, the world community has been alerted to the fact that we are living truly in the "radiation age." Each day our magazines, newspapers, radios, and television sets inform us about the health and environmental implication of radiation pollution, along the range of such different problems as microwaves, ultraviolet light and skin cancer, therapeutic and diagnostic x-rays, gamma irradiation of food, and nuclear fallout. As a consequence of this information, we often feel powerless, as if we can do nothing about the major source of this invisible, tasteless, odorless health robber called radiation. The book by Chaitow and Kutter helps to empower us with things we can do to combat the adverse effects of radiation. It is for this reason that this book, eloquently written in a style both readable and informative, makes such an important contribution to our libraries.

We first need to understand something about the physics and biology of radiation in order to properly defend ourselves against its adverse effects. We also need to be informed about what kind of environmental activism may be meaningful and what are both the short- and the long-term hazards associated with various forms of radiation exposure. We need to separate facts from fiction, myth from understanding, and fear from positive action. This book helps us to accomplish all of those goals. Clearly, the concept of radiation and health is a timely topic, but unfortunately it has been sensationalized too frequently. For this reason, this book is like a breath of fresh air, in that it incorporates accurate, substantive information along with understandable "how to" approaches toward protecting ourselves against radiation-induced health problems.

I recommend this book highly for readers who are trying to understand some of the complexities concerning radiation biology and the physiological significance of it, and want to know how to protect both themselves and the overall environment against both the short- and the long-term hazards of radiation.

JEFFREY S. BLAND, PH.D.
Nutritional Biochemist
President
HealthComm, Inc.

HOW TO LIVE
WITH LOW-LEVEL
RADIATION

CHAPTER ONE

RADIATION AND ITS EFFECTS

Life on earth has always been exposed to radiation from a variety of earthly and cosmic sources. In a sense, the very existence of life as we know it is owed to the effects of radiation, since the genetic changes which are key to the process of evolution are often triggered by the influence of radiation on the DNA of which the genes of all plants, animals, and humans are made.

These same radiation-induced mutations can, however, be of substantial concern when they are induced at high rates, potentially leading to cancer, birth defects, and premature aging. Thus, much of Europe watched with a sense of helplessness and panic as the invisible cloud of radioactive material released by the explosion at Chernobyl wafted in capricious, wind-driven fashion in its direction — radiation equal to the total that had been released to date by all of the bombs and weapons testing, hundreds of times that released at Hiroshima and Nagasaki, but much less localized! How much danger was there, in fact, at the levels people were encountering, and what could and should people be doing to protect themselves? The answers from different sources varied enormously, reflecting our ignorance as well as political exigencies. The main purpose of this book is empowerment: to help people obtain the knowledge base necessary for making wise decisions, to the degree that this is possible with our current understanding of the factors influencing radiation effects.

Chernobyl was the accident that most people in the field had claimed never could happen; it reflected an almost unbelievable series of events showing blatant lack of understanding of—and disregard for—safety considerations. We all may hope that the lessons learned will never be forgotten and that there will never be another Chernobyl—or another war involving nuclear weapons. However, people will still be continually exposed to radiation from many sources, such as these:

- the long-lasting fallout from Chernobyl, still present throughout much of Europe and the Ukraine,

- therapeutic or diagnostic radiation treatments or conducting research using radioisotopes,

- the radioactive lead and polonium often found in cigarette smoke,

- radon gas leaking into homes from the bedrock,

- the occasional venting necessary at nuclear power plants, and the cleanup jobs in decommissioning and decontaminating such plants, and

- cosmic rays, which are the emissions from our "major nuclear plant," the sun, and other stellar sources.

We explore here the evidence indicating that nutritional measures can, indeed, substantially limit the degree of damage resulting from very high-level radiation exposure. Only at high levels are the consequences extensive and obvious enough to enable reasonable assessment of such effects. Many of the resulting precautions and suggestions should be applicable also to long-term exposure to low-level ionizing radiation, but very few direct data are available on the effects of this radiation. The situation is in many ways parallel to trying to determine the ability to cause cancer, or *carcinogenicity,* of any substance; the saccharin debate is a case in point. The experiments and detailed studies have to be done at relatively high doses, where there are sufficient effects in most individuals to achieve statistically meaningful results without using impossibly large numbers of subjects. But critics of these studies can then claim that the results are irrelevant to the real situation, in which people are exposed to very low levels for long times. The results to date indicate that generally such data can, indeed, be extrapolated down to quite low dosage levels. This implies that for radiation, as for most other carcinogens, there is no *threshold* – no safe level of exposure below which *no* harm is done. Thus, the information presented here should help you make better, more informed decisions about protection from low-level exposure, as well as being an important resource in the unwelcome eventuality of high-level exposure.

Most of the basic principles we will examine turn out, in fact, simply to be an extension of those practices found by the National Academy of Sciences National Research Council to be generally associated with a lower overall risk of developing cancer, as described in its book *Diet, Nutrition and Cancer*. Because the same general principles also apply to improving our ability to withstand most other toxic materials in our environment, many of which have effects similar to those of radiation, it is sensible to incorporate these into our daily practice.

One complication in developing strategies for protection from radiation is that there are many different kinds of radiation and radioactive materials, deriving from a multitude of sources. These have various abilities to penetrate the body and to affect different parts of the body. In this chapter, we will first try to develop a basic understanding of the different kinds of radiation, with particular emphasis on *ionizing* radiation, which is responsible for most of the damage to our cells. We will look at the types of damage from different kinds of ionizing radiation, and attempt to make some sense out of the complex job of describing radiation strengths, given these variations. Much of this material, while challenging, provides the reader with scientific information to refer back to as needed. Chapter 2 uses the basic concepts developed in the first chapter to examine the concept of *free radicals*, the primary radiation products in our bodies (and also the direct causes of much of the damage from smoking and chemical pollutants). Luckily, as is explored in detail in Chapter 3, there is good evidence suggesting that nutritional practices can substantially reduce free-radical damage during exposure. Chapter 4 deals with additional, more general approaches to reducing radiation damage and enhancing repair, and Chapter 5 makes specific suggestions for applying the concepts of Chapters 3 and 4 in preparation for radiation therapy. Chapter 6 deals with the special problems of radioactive materials in our bodies, and ways to block their entry and enhance their removal. Finally, Chapter

7 summarizes the various sources of radiation to which we may be exposed, with particular suggestions as to precautions.

DIFFERENT TYPES OF RADIATION

When we speak of radiation, we should be aware that there are two very different types. The first general class consists of actual *physical particles,* such as electrons or the nuclei of helium atoms, which are ejected at high speed by radioactive atoms. These so-called "beta" and "alpha" rays will be discussed in a later section.

The second general class, called *electromagnetic radiation,* includes a continuous spectrum of "light" ranging from cosmic rays and x-rays through ultraviolet (UV) and visible light to microwaves and radio waves; all of them are basically the same, differing only in energy, strange though that may seem to many of us. The most energetic of them—the cosmic, gamma, and x-rays—are called *ionizing radiation,* as are the alpha and beta rays just mentioned. This name reflects the ability of such radiation to inflict heavy damage on atoms with which it collides, as will be described in more detail. The main focus of this book is on these two categories of ionizing radiation. Nonionizing electromagnetic radiation, such as radio waves and visible light, also have been suggested to have strong effects on living organisms, but the mechanisms are almost certainly quite different. Rather than damaging individual cells and molecules, they probably exert their effects more subtly on normal processes in the organism.

What, exactly, is the difference between these different kinds of electromagnetic radiation? To put it differently, how does an x-ray differ from visible light and from microwaves? After years of debate and confusion, it was finally determined early in this century that electromagnetic radiation actually must be described in two apparently contradictory ways at the same time: as minute particles and as waves. All forms of electromagnetic rays consist of enormously large numbers of exceedingly small entities called *photons,* which have virtually no mass. In a vacuum, these photons travel at the speed of light (186,000 miles per second), slowing somewhat in liquid or air. However, paradoxically, these "particles" move in a wavelike manner, like a series of ocean swells spaced at very precise distances rather

Figure 1.
Radiation wavelengths.

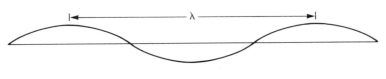

than like discrete particles. The kind of radiation, its energy, and thus its physical effects depend solely on the distance between successive wave crests, or the *wavelength* (λ) of the radiation (Figure 1). This radiation can also be characterized by its *frequency*, or the number of waves passing any point each second. For any kind of wave, the longer the wavelength, the shorter the frequency, but the product of the frequency and the wavelength is equal to the speed with which the waves move. Thus, for electromagnetic radiation, the frequency times the wavelength equals the speed of light, so we can specify either frequency or wavelength: knowing one, we can calculate the other. The wavelengths vary over an amazingly wide range, from about 0.000000000001 inch for cosmic rays to 100,000 inches, or nearly 2 miles, for radio waves.

The energy of electromagnetic radiation depends on the form of the wave. The higher the frequency—or the shorter the wavelength—the higher the energy, and thus, also, the greater the penetrating power and destructive potential.

Figure 2 gives the whole scale of electromagnetic energy, indicating also the sizes of certain relevant structures on the scale of wavelength. The dividing line between ionizing and nonionizing radiation is also indicated in Figure 2. At the boundary between the two comes ultraviolet radiation, which, while not ionizing, has its own very specific potential for causing damage, owing to its highly specific interaction, discussed later, with the DNA of our genes; this is why, for example, too much sunlight can cause skin cancer.

In order to go further in our understanding of ionizing radiation, we need next to take a basic look at the structure of atoms and how it relates to both the production of ionizing radiation and the ways in which it causes damage. These next few sections are the most technical of the book, but they are

Figure 2.
Scale of electromagnetic energy.

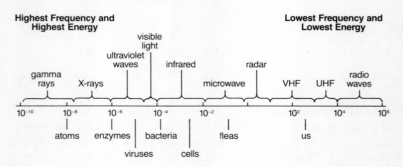

SIZE IN CENTIMETERS OF VARIOUS OBJECTS AND RADIATION WAVELENGTHS

essential to an understanding of the whole concept of radiation effects.

ATOMS, MOLECULES AND RADIOACTIVE DECAY

Everything in the universe is made up of combinations of about a hundred basic *elements*, such as hydrogen, oxygen, carbon, and sulfur. The smallest unit of each of these elements is the *atom*, just as the smallest unit of our money system is the penny. Each atom can be thought of as a tiny solar system. At the center is the *nucleus*. The nucleus contains *positively* charged particles called *protons*; the *number* of these protons it contains determines what element—what kind of atom—it is. For example, hydrogen always has only one proton in its nucleus, carbon has six, oxygen has eight, sodium has 11, calcium has 20, and uranium has 92. *Thus, the number of protons determines each atom's chemical properties, including its interactions in our bodies.*

The "planets" in the atomic solar systems are the *electrons*. They are *negatively* charged, each exactly balancing the positive charge of one proton, so an atom has exactly as many electrons as protons and is therefore neutral. The electrons are much smaller—it would take 1,835 electrons to equal one proton in weight—and they are constantly moving, like hyperactive children. Electrons have two other properties that are very important for our discussion here:

1. Like most people, they very strongly prefer to live in pairs. In fact, the "free radicals" mentioned earlier, which are responsible for most radiation damage, are actually just molecules with unpaired electrons.

2. In addition, the electrons are arranged in *shells*, which stay at definite distances from the nucleus, rather like the planets in our solar system. Each shell can hold only a certain number of electrons: the first two electrons go into the shell closest to the nucleus, then eight can go into each of the next two shells, and so on. (The outermost shells of very heavy atoms get a bit more complex, but similar principles apply.)

Thus, *two* sets of forces affect the number of electrons in a given atom. (1) As in the rest of nature, there is a push to be electrically neutral—since positive and negative charges attract each other—which is manifested here in having the same number of electrons and protons in each atom. (2) Sometimes the pressure to have complete families, or shells, is in competition with the need to be neutral. The action of these two factors simultaneously is what leads some kinds of atoms to *share* electrons with other atoms so that they become bonded together to form *molecules*, like water or sugar. Other atoms find it easier to lose or gain from one to three electrons to make charged *ions*, which then interact loosely with each other in complex *arrays* to neutralize the charges.

For example, a sodium atom has 11 protons, so it must also have 11 electrons; its first two electrons go into the first shell, eight more go into the next, and this leaves only one so-called "valence" electron in the outermost shell. That electron is very easily lost to any passing atom that needs just one electron to complete a shell, such as chlorine, which has 17 protons and 17 electrons; there are two and eight electrons in the inner shells and only seven in its outermost shell. The sodium atom, symbolized Na, then becomes a positively charged sodium ion, symbolized Na^+, while the chlorine atom (Cl) becomes a negatively charged chloride ion, Cl^-. (See example, next page.)

Enormous numbers of sodium and chloride ions then interact with each other in regular arrays to form each crystal of the substance we know as table salt (sodium chloride).

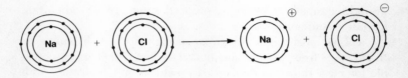

The *periodic table*, shown on page nine, shows all of the elements arranged in order by number of protons, or *atomic number*. Each *row* represents the filling of one of the shells, so there are two elements in the first row and eight each in the next two. Elements (atoms) in the same vertical *column* have similar chemical properties. These relationships will be important as we talk in Chapter 6 about dealing with actual radioactive materials.

RADIOACTIVITY

Most atoms are very stable, lasting forever. However, there are some that are *unstable*, or *radioactive*, and spontaneously change into other atoms while giving off a great deal of energy in a form so intense that it is capable of knocking electrons out of other atoms and molecules. Since the result is to create an ion—a charged atom or molecule—the radiation released from radioactive atoms is called *ionizing radiation*. Such ionizing radiation often leaves a whole path of havoc, each particle bouncing from molecule to molecule until all its energy is spent, causing serious damage to biological molecules such as DNA and membrane lipids and providing the main concern in dealing with radioactive materials.

Just what makes some atoms radioactive? In addition to protons, atoms have one other kind of particle in the nucleus, called *neutrons*. Neutrons are as big as protons, and thus are just as important in determining the actual weight of the atom, but they have no electrical charge. Each kind of atom, each element, can be found in nature in several different forms, called *isotopes* of the element, which have different numbers of neutrons. For example, most hydrogen atoms have only a proton in their nuclei, but two rare forms of hydrogen, deuterium and tritium, are isotopes with one and two neutrons, respectively, in addition to the single proton.

Isotopes—both stable and unstable—are designated by the standard symbol for the element (found in the periodic table)

Figure 3.
The periodic table.

IA	IIA	IIIB	IVB	VB	VIB	VIIB	VIIIB	VIIIB	VIIIB	IB	IIB	IIIA	IVA	VA	VIA	VIIA	VIII
1 **H** Hydrogen 1.01																	2 **He** Helium 4.00
3 **Li** Lithium 6.94	4 **Be** Beryllium 9.01											5 **B** Boron 10.8	6 **C** Carbon 12.0	7 **N** Nitrogen 14.0	8 **O** Oxygen 16.0	9 **F** Fluorine 19.0	10 **Ne** Neon 20.2
11 **Na** Sodium 23.0	12 **Mg** Magnesium 24.3											13 **Al** Aluminum 27.0	14 **Si** Silicon 28.1	15 **P** Phosphorus 31.0	16 **S** Sulfur 32.1	17 **Cl** Chlorine 35.5	18 **Ar** Argon 39.9
19 **K** Potassium 39.1	20 **Ca** Calcium 40.1	21 **Sc** Scandium 45.0	22 **Ti** Titanium 47.9	23 **V** Vanadium 51.0	24 **Cr** Chromium 52.0	25 **Mn** Manganese 54.9	26 **Fe** Iron 55.9	27 **Co** Cobalt 58.9	28 **Ni** Nickel 58.7	29 **Cu** Copper 63.5	30 **Zn** Zinc 65.4	31 **Ga** Gallium 69.7	32 **Ge** Germanium 72.6	33 **As** Arsenic 74.9	34 **Se** Selenium 79.0	35 **Br** Bromine 79.9	36 **Kr** Krypton 83.8
37 **Rb** Rubidium 85.5	38 **Sr** Strontium 87.6	39 **Y** Yttrium 88.9	40 **Zr** Zirconium 91.2	41 **Nb** Niobium 92.9	42 **Mo** Molybdenum 95.9	43 **Tc** Technetium 98.9	44 **Ru** Ruthenium 101.1	45 **Rh** Rhodium 102.9	46 **Pd** Palladium 106.4	47 **Ag** Silver 107.9	48 **Cd** Cadmium 112	49 **In** Indium 115	50 **Sn** Tin 119	51 **Sb** Antimony 122	52 **Te** Tellurium 128	53 **I** Iodine 127	54 **Xe** Xenon 131
55 **Cs** Cesium 133	56 **Ba** Barium 137	57 **La** Lanthanum 139	72 **Hf** Hafnium 178	73 **Ta** Tantalum 181	74 **W** Tungsten 184	75 **Re** Rhenium 186	76 **Os** Osmium 190	77 **Ir** Iridium 192	78 **Pt** Platinum 195	79 **Au** Gold 197	80 **Hg** Mercury 201	81 **Tl** Thallium 204	82 **Pb** Lead 207	83 **Bi** Bismuth 209	84 **Po** Polonium (209)	85 **At** Astatine (210)	86 **Rn** Radon (222)
87 **Fr** Francium (223)	88 **Ra** Radium 226	89 **Ac** Actinium (227)	104 **Rf** Rutherfordium (261)	105 **Ha** Hahnium (262)													

58 **Ce** Cerium 140.1	59 **Pr** Praseodymium 140.9	60 **Nd** Neodymium 144.2	61 **Pm** Promethium (147)	62 **Sm** Samarium 150.3	63 **Eu** Europium 152.0	64 **Gd** Gadolinium 157.2	65 **Tb** Terbium 158.9	66 **Dy** Dysprosium 162.5	67 **Ho** Holmium 164.9	68 **Er** Erbium 167.3	69 **Tm** Thulium 168.9	70 **Yb** Ytterbium 173.0	71 **Lu** Lutecium 175.0
90 **Th** Thorium 232.0	91 **Pa** Protactinium 231.0	92 **U** Uranium 238.0	93 **Np** Neptunium 237.0	94 **Pu** Plutonium (242)	95 **Am** Americium (243)	96 **Cm** Curium (247)	97 **Bk** Berkelium (247)	98 **Cf** Californium (251)	99 **Es** Einsteinium (254)	100 **Fm** Fermium (253)	101 **Md** Mendelevium (256)	102 **No** Nobelium (254)	103 **Lr** Lawrencium (257)

with a superscript number giving the *atomic weight* of that isotope: the total number of protons plus neutrons in its nucleus.
Tritium is denoted ^{3}H, and some other important radioisotopes
are ^{14}C (read "carbon 14"), ^{32}P (phosphorus 32), ^{131}I (iodine
131), and ^{137}Cs (cesium 137).

For some reason, each kind of atom has a preferred *ratio* of
protons to neutrons, usually somewhere near one. If the atom
starts out at too high or low a ratio, it undergoes the profound
changes we call *radioactive decay* to move toward that balance.
This may happen slowly or rapidly, over seconds or centuries;
the rate is a fixed characteristic for that particular kind of atom. It
is measured in terms of a *half-life*, defined as the time it takes for
half of the atoms to undergo the change. For each individual
atom, you can never tell when the change will actually happen;
but after one half-life, half of the radioactive material will be left;
after two half-lives, a quarter will be left; after three half-lives, an
eighth, and so forth. Those isotopes that are unstable are called
radioisotopes, reflecting their ability to undergo radioactive decay. For instance, ordinary hydrogen and deuterium (with one
proton and one neutron) are both stable, but tritium (with one
proton and two neutrons) is a radioisotope that has a half-life of
about 10 years.

Radioactive decay can release any of three different kinds of
ionizing radiation, and the nature and severity of the damage it
can do depend on both the kind of radiation released and how
energetic it is. These are both specific characteristics of each
kind of radioisotope. The three kinds of radiation are these:

1. *Alpha.* A large nucleus like that of uranium 238 can lose
two neutrons and two protons simultaneously as a single particle.
This is called an *alpha* (α) particle. It usually doesn't penetrate
very far through biological materials, but it leaves a very dense,
intense path of havoc as it goes. Atoms which decay in this
fashion can particularly cause problems if they are inhaled or
eaten.

2. *Beta.* A neutron is able to decay into a proton, which stays
in the nucleus, plus an electron, which shoots out of the nucleus
at very high speed. These high-energy ejected electrons are
called *beta* (β) particles. Their energy ranges from that of the
beta particles ejected during decay of tritium or ^{14}C, which
doesn't even penetrate the skin, to that of ^{32}P or ^{131}I, which can
penetrate glass and can travel far enough internally to cause

considerable damage. A number of the isotopes which decay in this fashion are atoms which can become incorporated into biological molecules, remaining in the body and leading to particular problems when they decay. An example is the decay of carbon 14:

$$^{14}C \rightarrow {}^{14}N + e^- \text{ (beta)}$$

Here, one either may end up with a nitrogen where there should be a carbon in the molecule or may have a bond next to the carbon broken in the process, as well as having the beta particle shoot off to cause damage elsewhere.

3. *Gamma.* In many cases of radioactive decay, energy is also released in the form of *gamma* (γ) rays, which are pure electromagnetic radiation, similar to x-rays, as discussed earlier. For example, they also are able to penetrate solid material, with the degree of penetration and damage depending on their spectrum of wavelengths and thus their energy. This, in turn, is characteristic of the particular isotope that is undergoing decay.

When a heavy radioisotope such as uranium 235 is bombarded with energetic neutrons, as in a power plant or nuclear explosion, it can also fragment or explode into various large pieces, some of which may themselves be radioactive and continue to decay further (Figure 4). This is where the dangerous ^{131}I and strontium 90 came from in the Chernobyl explosion, for example, or in the fallout from nuclear tests.

How Do We Actually Measure the Amount of Radiation Present?

Since we can't see radiation or radioactivity, how do we know that it is there? The measurement of radioactivity involves adaptations of the methods used in measuring other kinds of light. Various common methods differ in sensitivity and in their ability to detect different kinds of radiation, with different energies. It is important to be aware that any discussion of the amount of radioactivity present is thus limited by the methods used to detect the radiation. Such methods include the following:

Film badges, used to monitor exposure of workers to hazardous radiation, are simply pieces of x-ray film in special little packets that can be pinned on the jacket and taken out and developed regularly. Any radiation energetic enough to penetrate the clothes and skin and cause internal damage will also

Figure 4.
A fission chain reaction.

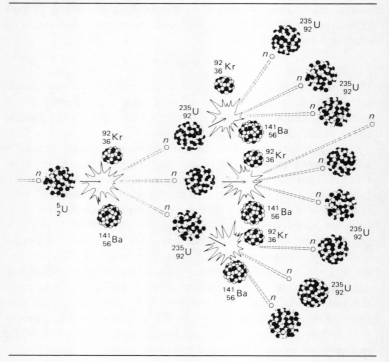

expose the x-ray film, but the badges don't pick up those kinds of radioisotopes which are harmful only if they are ingested into our bodies.

Geiger counters are the detectors commonly sold for the private monitoring of radiation. A kind of photomultiplier tube, with a meter attached, is pointed at the area to be checked. Radiation entering the tube strikes special detectors, where it momentarily creates an electric response, and the resulting signal is then amplified enough to generate a little current of electricity and move a needle on a meter. Just as the volume control on a stereo receiver can be set to get different amounts of amplification of the input from the recording, there are different settings on the Geiger counter scale to give different sensitivities and allow quantitative measurement over a wide range of radiation levels. The output is in the form of *counts per minute* (cpm), which is generally proportional to the actual number of radioactive decays, or *disintegrations per minute* (dpm). However, only radiation energetic enough to get through the window of the probe and activate the detectors can be measured; thus, the Geiger counter is fairly efficient for measuring the very energetic decay of iodine 131 but doesn't pick up the weak radiation from tritium at all.

Scintillation counters are very complex, expensive devices, used in laboratories, which permit the measurement of all kinds of radioisotopes with reasonable efficiency as long as a sample can be put into the machine. The name comes from the use of materials that emit a minute scintillation of light when they absorb the energy of a decaying radioisotope. These devices can even be used to identify the different kinds of radioisotopes in a sample by carefully analyzing the spectrum of energy which is being produced.

How Do We Describe Radiation Strengths?

This subject is unavoidably very complicated. There are two main concerns in measuring radioactive material. First, how much radioactivity is actually present? Second, how much of an effect will this have on the material it strikes—specifically, on us? Since the *effect* on us is very much dependent on the *nature* and *energy* of the radiation as well as the *amount*, there is no general or straightforward relationship between these two kinds of measures, and quite different sets of units are used. Furthermore, the units themselves are complicated for historical reasons, just as there are no simple relationships between the inch, the yard, and the mile.

The total *amount* of radioactive material present is measured in either *curies* or, recently, *becquerels*. The curie is named after Marie Curie, who in 1898 began studying the radiation given off by materials like radium, coining the term "radioactivity" and devoting her life to discovering and distinguishing between alpha, beta, and gamma rays. A curie (Ci) is a very large unit: the amount of radiation given off by 1 gram of pure radium 286, which corresponds to 37 billion atoms, disintegrating per second. This unit is so big that the amount of radioactive material is more often expressed in millicuries (mCi) or microcuries (μCi), corresponding to 37 million or 37,000 disintegrations per second, respectively. Recently, a far smaller unit was introduced (reflecting in part our increasing ability to measure very low levels of radioactivity). One *becquerel* is defined as one atom disintegrating per second. It is named after the actual discoverer of radioactivity; in 1896, Antoine Henri Becquerel, a professor at the Ecole Polytechnique in Paris, discovered that uranium emits an invisible radiation which in many ways resembles roentgen rays (what we now call x-rays) and which can cloud a photographic plate after passing through thin plates of metal.

The measurement of the effective radiation dose received is even more complex. The same units are used whether we are talking about electromagnetic radiation or about particles such as alpha or beta rays: roentgens, rad, and rem, or more recently, grays. The *roentgen* is a physical unit, used particularly to quantify outputs, as for x-ray machines, and says nothing about the actual nature of the material in the path. It is also termed the *effective dose delivered* by the radiation at a given spot in space and is a measure of *exposure* to a particular form of radiation. Its definition is rather complex: 1 roentgen is the amount of radiation that produces 2 billion ions in 1 cubic centimeter of air under standard conditions, so it is quite a large unit.

This measure of *delivered* radiation does not take into account the interaction of radiation with different tissues. For this purpose, *biological* units are also needed. The amount of radiation actually *absorbed* by a given part of the body is expressed in *rad* (radiation absorbed dose), called also *rem* (radiation equivalent in man) when referring specifically to human exposure. These are measures of the effect on a given piece of tissue of exposure to 1 roentgen of radiation. One roentgen is generally equal to between 0.9 and 3 rad, depending on the kind of radiation and the kind of tissue involved. (It is this differential effect in different tissues that, for example, makes x-ray photographs possible; the bone absorbs much more of the radiation than does the soft tissue, thus casting a shadow on the plate.) The *gray* and the *sievert* are two new units of measurement sometimes used in place of the rad and the rem to describe the level of radiation absorbed by various parts of the body. One gray is defined as one joule of energy deposited per kilogram of tissue; one gray is equal to 100 rad. One sievert is similarly equal to 100 rem.

The effects from various kinds of radiation differ. One rad

Figure 5.
Radiation exposure to the average U.S. citizen—
between 100 and 200 millirems per year.

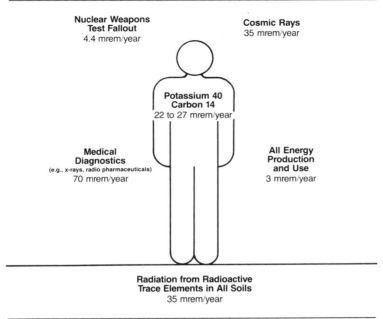

**Nuclear Weapons
Test Fallout**
4.4 mrem/year

Cosmic Rays
35 mrem/year

**Potassium 40
Carbon 14**
22 to 27 mrem/year

**Medical
Diagnostics**
(e.g., x-rays, radio pharmaceuticals)
70 mrem/year

**All Energy
Production
and Use**
3 mrem/year

**Radiation from Radioactive
Trace Elements in All Soils**
35 mrem/year

from alpha rays or neutrons, for example, causes ten times more damage than 1 rad from x-rays or gamma rays to a given amount of tissue. However, alpha particles have very low penetrating power and cannot even pass through the skin, so they actually can do no harm unless they get inside the body and are incorporated into tissue.

How Much Exposure Is a Rem?

From various natural sources, all of us are exposed to about 0.1 rem per year whole body radiation. This number gets larger at higher altitudes, as in Denver, where it is about 0.15 rem. Also there are areas where substantial natural radioactivity is present from radon released within the bedrock, as well as from natural deposits of uranium.

Figure 5 shows the levels of radiation exposure from various sources encountered by the average U.S. citizen each year.

A radiograph of a broken arm would add about 0.02 rem (also expressed as 20 millirem, or mrem). For chest radiographs, the precise value depends on the skill of the operator as well as the functioning of the machine; the average is about 50 mrem. A gastrointestinal tract diagnostic series delivers about 2 rem. Recent United States guidelines suggest that persons over 18 should receive an exposure of not over 300 mrem per week with no more than a total of 5 rem per year. Young children are far more vulnerable, and radiation levels should be kept much lower for them.

In United States power stations, workers are advised to receive no more than 3 rem per 3 months; the average such worker receives only about 0.15. A similar figure holds for the average airline pilot.

Doses of about 25 rem produce notable blood changes. Above 100 rem of whole body radiation, signs of radiation sickness begin to appear: fatigue, weakness, loss of appetite, nausea, vomiting, skin changes, loss of hair, and gastrointestinal problems. Most of these are reversible. At about 400 rem, half of the exposed people generally die, and death is virtually certain after exposure to a dose above 600 rem, unless extraordinary measures are taken to replace the bone marrow.

Microorganisms are far less sensitive; about 50,000 rem are needed to reliably kill bacteria, as in food irradiation. The lethal dose for insects is also far greater than that for people.

What Parts of Our Bodies Are Most Vulnerable?

Radiation can cause damage to virtually any of the molecules of which our cells are made; the major mechanisms are discussed in the next chapter. However, our cells have also evolved many kinds of repair mechanisms, and most of the individual molecules in each cell are continually being replaced: the enzymes that carry out cell function, the fats and proteins that make up the membrane that surrounds each cell, the ribosomes that act as factories for protein synthesis, and the messenger RNA that directs that synthesis. However, one part of every cell is irreplaceable: the DNA that carries the information directing and controlling all of these processes. Thus, the major form of damage that can lead to long-term cell malfunction and/or cancer is damage to the DNA, which is particularly susceptible to free-radical effects because of both its composition and its shape. The other potentially serious kind of damage, even on a short-term basis, is damage to cell membranes, interfering with cell–cell communication and with maintaining the proper balance between the substances that belong inside the cell and the substances that belong outside. These are discussed in more detail in Chapter 4.

On a larger scale, the parts of our body that are most vulnerable are those where the cells are dividing most rapidly—those that have the least chance to carry out repair before having to repeatedly grow and divide. Thus, the cells and organs where radiation damage is most apparent and problematic are the immune system, the gastrointestinal tract, and the skin. These are, of course, also our chief lines of defense against outside infection, and the latter two are crucial in maintaining proper internal composition, rendering us particularly vulnerable and particularly in need of optimum nutritional support.

CHAPTER TWO

FREE RADICALS:
The Consequences
of Oxidation

In order to see just what antiradiation benefits are available from nutritional sources, we need to look at the ways in which radiation causes damage within our bodies. The major tissue effects to be considered are those from so-called *free radicals* and highly reactive *oxidation products*.

Much of the damage we will discuss here is some kind of *oxidation*. Oxidation is commonly the addition of oxygen atoms to some other atom or molecule. For instance, rusting is an oxidation process in which iron atoms (Fe) are combined with oxygen to make an iron oxide, such as Fe_2O_3. While oxygen is an important component of most of the organic molecules of our cells and tissues, it can also create great damage. It may seem paradoxical that oxygen, the stuff we depend on for life, can also be a poison, but in the wrong amounts and at the wrong place it certainly is.

Ionizing radiation is, by definition, able to knock individual electrons out of atoms and molecules, leaving behind a *single, unpaired* electron on the molecule; it is this highly reactive form of any molecule which is called a *free radical* or, at times, a *free oxidizing radical* (for). As discussed in Chapter 1, electrons have a very strong preference for being in pairs, so this free radical bounces around, creating havoc in other molecules, until it finally finds a new partner and settles down. Most free radicals are thus quickly inactivated, with a half-life of only milliseconds. However, the oxygen molecule (O_2) is so reactive and potentially damaging because it most frequently exists as a rather stable *double* free radical, with unpaired electrons on each end. It is this characteristic which also makes O_2 interact so readily with other free radicals, forming activated peroxides. Del Maestro (1980) presents an excellent discussion of these issues.

SOURCES OF FREE RADICALS

Ionizing radiation is by no means the only source of free radicals and highly reactive derivatives of oxygen in our bodies. Many are formed as intermediates (transiently) in the normal course of cell function, and must be dealt with continually by the cells. Others are produced as a consequence of carbon monoxide, pesticides, smog, and exhaust fumes. Consider the effect on the eyes of being in an area where there is a high level of atmospheric pollution. They start to sting and soon become watery and irritated. This is mainly the effect on the eye surface of free radical activity. The tears carry away the free radicals, and this largely relieves the stinging and smarting effects, although there may be some lingering damage. The mucous membranes of the nose, throat, and lungs can be similarly affected by inhaling the free radicals in polluted air, causing a runny nose, inflamed sinuses, and coughing of protective mucus from the lungs. The fumes from fresh paint or dry cleaning, and a host of chemicals in daily use in homes, offices, and industry are highly charged with oxidants and free radicals, and their oxidizing activity can be increased through activation by solar energy.

Sunburn also results from free radicals, in an unusual fashion that is rather intriguing and may help the reader visualize how such damage can happen. No ionizing radiation is involved. However, the ultraviolet rays of the sun interact with the red oxygen-carrying blood-cell pigment, hemoglobin, in areas near the skin surface, and they excite an electron on the oxygen (bound to the hemoglobin) to a more active state. Although still part of the oxygen molecule, the electron is then excited enough to interact with certain other molecules, such as membrane lipids, and cause the extensive damage we know as sunburn.

This is a fairly slow process, taking several hours, which is why we often don't realize we're burned until it is too late. Both this same process affecting DNA and direct DNA damage from ultraviolet (UV) light contribute to skin cancer. Tobacco smoke is a major offender. While most free radicals are very short-lived, interacting and disappearing in a very small fraction of a second, certain of the tobacco tar free radicals survive and can do damage for several days. (See Borish and Pryor [1987] for further discussion.) In addition, both carbon monoxide and nitrogen oxide are produced, which can help oxidize body fats. Tobacco smoke also contains hundreds of different compounds which are potentially toxic producers of free radicals and oxidation products.

Foods also can contribute to free-radical production. The rancidity of oil or whole-grain flour results from its accumulating oxidation products, affecting taste as well as nutritional quality. Even oxygen itself is very reactive; our cells have to go to great lengths to protect themselves and make sure that the "burning" of sugar and other nutrients—which provides the energy with which we operate—occurs in a controlled, stepwise fashion, capturing most of the energy in a useful chemical form, rather than in a destructive fashion, and that there is never much free oxygen sitting around.

Many of our white blood cells routinely make reactive molecules such as hydrogen peroxide and superoxide and use them to kill and digest bacteria and other garbage that they have ingested (taken in). However, this process is normally limited to special little sacks inside the cells, the *lysosomes*. (When tissue is injured so badly that some of these get outside the cells, substantial damage to normal tissue can happen, as in the inflammation process around a wound.) However, no such compartmentalization is there to protect us from radiation effects. For most pollutants that cause free-radical damage, only a relatively small fraction actually gets *into* the cells, where they can cause the most problems. In the case of radiation, on the other hand, many of the free radicals are actually being *produced* behind our defensive lines, as it were, making it even more important that all our intracellular antioxidants and free-radical scavengers function optimally to stop them before crucial molecules are damaged.

MECHANISMS OF RADIATION-INDUCED
FREE RADICAL DAMAGE

Our bodies are mainly water, and the major damage is actually caused by the products made when ionizing radiation strikes water. The water molecule, made of two hydrogen atoms bonded to one oxygen atom (H_2O), breaks down into a hydrogen ion (H^+), a fast-moving electron, e^-, and a *hydroxyl free radical, OH·*. (The OH group is called hydroxyl, and the dot is used to represent the very energetic unpaired electron.) A chemist would write this in shorthand:

$$H_2O \rightarrow e^- + H^+ + OH·$$

The fast-moving electron, in turn, can interact with other water molecules to release a hydrogen free radical, H., along with a negative hydroxyl ion, OH·. It also can collide with oxygen to form the highly reactive *superoxide anion, O_2^-*, which we will discuss later as the specific target of the enzyme SOD, or superoxide dismutase. Two other kinds of reactions happen to make a potentially destructive cascade:

$$2\ OH· \rightarrow HOOH$$

(This is hydrogen peroxide—and you know what it does to hair or clothes as bleach!)

$$H· + O_2 \rightarrow HOO·$$

(This is the reactive hydroperoxyl radical.)

These compounds, and several others made in similar fashion, very readily interact with so-called *double bonds* in membrane lipids, DNA molecules, and virtually anything else in the cell. (Normal single bonds in molecules are formed when two atoms share a pair of electrons; in a double bond, the same pair of atoms shares *two* pairs of electrons, and these electron pairs are more exposed and more vulnerable to attack by free radicals and oxidants than they are in single bonds.)

As you can see, having free radicals around is rather like having a bull loose in the china shop.

INTERACTION OF FREE RADICALS WITH CELL MEMBRANES AND SIMILAR MOLECULES

In a way, each of our cells is a miniature creature, with functions of its own and, in many cases, the ability to reproduce itself exactly. The outer "skin," within which the life of the cell is carried out, is called the *cell membrane*. It must be not only strong but capable of allowing the selective passage into the cell of the nutrients required for their function, including oxygen, which is needed to release energy from our food. It also controls the passage outward of waste materials. Furthermore, in it are embedded receptors which detect specific "signal" molecules and thus determine most aspects of the cell's interaction with the rest of the body. For example, specific membrane receptor proteins receive most of the hormonal and neurochemical messages from outside the cell and translate and amplify them to permit them to modulate cell function. Other receptors help keep the cell growing at the right rate and in the proper places in our bodies. In addition, the inside of the cell has a whole network of specialized membranes involved in deriving energy from sugars and fats, preparing proteins for export, detoxifying drugs, or making other processes more efficient.

Cell membranes are constructed mainly of special fats and cholesterol, which are particularly vulnerable to free-radical damage; in fact, approximately one molecule of vitamin E per 1,000 lipid (fat) molecules is normally present in the membrane, presumably to help protect against damage. The cell normally repairs these membranes constantly, slipping in new molecules here and there for repair and growth while slipping out old damaged ones. However, when a cell is exposed to high levels of radiation, where damage greatly exceeds the rate of repair, there may be substantial problems.

The reactions can be quite complex. For example, a peroxide radical may pull a hydrogen off a lipid molecule, leaving a lipid radical, which can now react with oxygen to form a lipid peroxide radical—a fatty chain which has an oxygen molecule stuck on its end with a reactive unpaired electron looking for trouble. This, in turn, can interact with another lipid molecule to produce a peroxidized lipid (one to which the oxygen molecule has been permanently attached, sometimes in the middle, causing the molecule to break in two in the process). At the same time it produces a new lipid radical which can begin the process all over again and carry on the chain.

The *polyunsaturated fatty acids* in the membrane lipids are the most vulnerable. These contain at least two closely spaced double bonds. Among these, the two families of essential fatty acids, omega-6 and omega-3, are particularly important; they and their roles are discussed in more detail in Chapter 4. Free radicals also attack the oxygen–oxygen bond of peroxides, making them more damaging. Radiation carcinogenesis from a membrane perspective is discussed in technical detail by Petkan (1980) and by Slater, Cheeseman, and Proudfoot (1984).

Sulfur-containing compounds are particularly good at protecting against radiation because they form disulfide bonds (bonds between two sulfur atoms, S–S), which are even more strongly attacked than the peroxide bonds, and molecules with SH groups can transfer the hydrogen atom to the lipid or other polymer radical, R. The resultant sulfur radical, R–S• (where R can be almost any group of atoms) is a good deal more stable and less lethal than most radicals. The reasons are beyond the scope of this discussion, but the consequence for our purposes is that such nutrients as methionine, cysteine, and glutathione have protective properties; these are discussed in the next chapter.

EFFECTS OF RADIATION AND FREE RADICALS ON DNA

DNA is the control center of each of our cells, the physical repository of our genetic information. Two kinds of effects on DNA have potentially very serious results for the cell: *chromosome breakage*, often followed by rejoining of the pieces in abnormal fashion, and *mutagenesis*, or changes in the information encoded in the cell.

Let us look more carefully at just what is happening. The information for each cell is arranged like the bits along a computer tape, in its 23 pairs of DNA molecules. An incredible number of "words," or bits of information, are involved: about 1 billion, or enough to fill 50 20-volume encyclopedias. Yet, the threads that carry all this crucial information are incredibly delicate. A piece of DNA long enough to reach from here to the sun would only weigh about half a gram! The DNA in each cell is a meter long if we put together the pieces from all of our chromosomes, and each of us has about 25 billion kilometers of DNA in our bodies.

This genetic code is written in a language of only four letters, which are the sub-units or components of the DNA. These four kinds of small molecules are called bases, and their names are abbreviated A, G, C, and T. In DNA, successive bases or "letters" are connected to each other along a backbone rather like beads on a string, with only a single, vulnerable bond connecting each bead to the next. However, one additional feature of DNA makes the information slightly less vulnerable and facilitates both its duplication during cell division and its repair under some circumstances. The DNA is actually present in the cell in the form of a *double helix*, made up of two parallel such strands; opposite each of the bases is a complementary base, A pairing with T, and G with C, so that each of the two strands has all the information and can serve as a template for resynthesis of the other in case of damage.

The major kind of information encoded in the DNA is that specifying the *sequence of amino acids* in each of the many thousands of proteins the cell is capable of making; here, a sequence of three nucleotides codes for each amino acid. In addition, some stretches of the DNA have various *control functions*, involved in regulating the *timing* and *extent* of synthesis of each of the possible proteins so that it will be appropriate for that particular kind of cell. There are also many parts of the DNA whose functions we don't yet know.

Radiation can directly break one or both strands of the DNA through hits direct on it or in its vicinity. Free radicals can cause damage by attacking either the bonds between units or the actual "letters" of the code themselves. There are repair enzymes that cut out altered nucleotides or the damaged bases next to a single-strand break, but an imperfect repair process sometimes leads to mutations as a consequence. These, in turn, may destroy the function of the gene or alter its regulation.

Double-strand breaks are particularly serious, since they

separate part of the DNA molecule from the rest of the chromosome. As well as potentially breaking into the middle of a gene or
its control sequence(s), this can destroy the fragment's ability, at
subsequent cell divisions, to properly provide copies to both
daughter cells. Alternatively, the broken ends may remain in a
somewhat activated, "sticky" state long enough to stick onto the
end of some other chromosome, possibly also a broken one.
This, in turn, can lead to production of a new, hybrid gene, or it
can drastically alter the proper control of expression of the gene,
leading to cancer, birth defects, or abnormal cell function.

MECHANISM OF RADIATION-INDUCED CARCINOGENESIS

Over the last few years, we have developed a much better
understanding of the ways in which *cancer* is caused, by radiation as well as by other carcinogens. This insight has come
primarily from the study of *viruses* that are able to cause cancer
in animals. Genetic engineering techniques have showed that
causing cancer doesn't involve the whole virus; in each case, only
one or two specific viral genes are needed to make cells grow in
excessive fashion. These genes, called *oncogenes,* were found to
be similar or identical to so-called *proto-oncogenes,* genes already
present in the host cell that are responsible for normal control
of cell growth and differentiation. Causing cancer was related
to altered forms or to gross overproduction of these regulatory
factors. About 30 different genes that have such potential have
now been identified.

   Radiation-induced carcinogenesis appears also to be due to
changes in the functioning of some of these proto-oncogenes.
The genes may be mutated by the radiation, or, more probably,
DNA breakage and rejoining may lead to putting the proto-
oncogene under the control of some other piece of DNA that
causes it to be expressed excessively and inappropriately, leading to excessive, poorly controlled rates of growth. Additional
later mutations, made more probable by the cells' increased
frequency of replication, are generally needed before a full-
blown cancer can develop, a fact that helps explain why many of
the effects of radiation are cumulative over time. Other factors
that affect the *rate* and *extent* of *cell growth* can also act to
promote cancer production, increasing the probability of an *al-*

ready initiated cancer developing into a problematic tumor. These promoters include various hormones, plant substances, nitrosamines, elements in tobacco smoke, and anything causing chronic tissue damage and repair. Radiation can also act as a promoter, through its effects on membranes and general tissue damage.

Only a very small fraction of radiation-induced mutations may have the potential to cause cancer, but many more may adversely affect cell function and/or lead to premature cell aging and death, or to the production of daughter cells with abnormal chromosome patterns. In the developing fetus, the potential for serious damage is particularly high. On the positive side, the majority of such mutations may well have no observable effect, occurring in stretches of the DNA that are inactive in that particular cell and its daughters or that do not destroy vital functions.

EFFECTS OF FREE RADICALS ON PROTEINS

Radiation can, in effect, cause premature aging of cells through damaging their proteins directly or affecting the machinery that makes them. However, turnover of most cellular enzymes is so rapid that this is not a serious long-term problem for most proteins as long as the information in the DNA is still intact. A significant problem occurs, however, in the case of the collagen that acts as the matrix of our connective tissue and is important in many aspects of tissue health, structure, and function. The free radicals interact with sulfur amino acids and cause the collagen fibers to become inappropriately cross-linked, adversely affecting tissue elasticity and ability to support other physiological functions.

EFFECTS ON SPECIFIC TISSUES

As mentioned in Chapter 1, rapidly dividing cells are particularly vulnerable to radiation effects, leading to many problems with white blood cells (leukemia and abnormal functioning), skin (sluffing, blistering, and melanoma) and the intestinal lining (sluffing, poor nutrient uptake, breakdown of its barrier function, and diarrhea). The lungs are particularly vulnerable, since they must also deal with very high oxygen levels, potentiating the direct effects of free radicals, and with the possibility of inhaled radioactive particles and other irritants. The heart is also made more vulnerable through its high oxygen tension and very high metabolic rate. On the other hand, the brain, with little cell division and high antioxidant levels is generally relatively unaffected. It is particularly vulnerable only in the fetus and the young infant, when very rapid cell division is taking place; other tissues are also much more sensitive at this stage. The ovum itself is very vulnerable since it has little antioxidant activity or repair and since virtually all of its genetic information is crucial in supplying the blueprint for the next generation.

The immune system is particularly vulnerable to radiation, as well, in the short term as well as the long term. One consequence of this in the general population seems to be increased general susceptibility to a wide variety of infectious agents during periods of increased radiation. Much of the evidence for this is reviewed by Sternglass (1986). One of the most striking examples which appears to be attributable to this cause is the strong correlation between the occurrence in New York City of epidemic encephalitis, which is generally quite rare, and atmospheric nuclear explosions (Figure 6). The effects seem to be detectable, though of course less dramatic, in a variety of other kinds of conditions, such as pneumonia, influenza, and general infant mortality. In these cases, we are talking about virtually *immediate* correlations rather than the long lag periods seen for carcinogenesis. It will be important to look for such potential correlations with the well-documented levels of exposure in various parts of Europe in the aftermath of Chernobyl to confirm that these apparent correlations indeed reflect the effects of relatively low-level radiation exposure.

We will talk directly in the next chapter about ways of enhancing the body's ability to inactivate free radicals and strong oxidants before they cause too much damage. However, it also makes sense to try to limit our exposure to other sources of free radicals during periods when we are being exposed to ionizing radiation, to allow our defense mechanisms to focus on the radiation damage. In particular, this includes such measures as avoiding the fumes of paints and organic chemicals, not smoking or being around smokers, avoiding polluted areas as much as possible, and avoiding foods fried in deep fat, cured meats and

Figure 6.
Number of cases of reported encephalitis per
1 million people in New York City, 1935–1970.

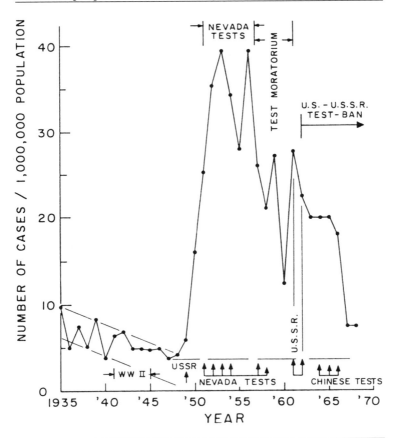

oils, or whole grains that may be rancid. It also means staying out
of the sun and avoiding contact in air, food, or water with such
heavy metals as lead, mercury, and cadmium, which also can
catalyze free-radical production.

CHAPTER THREE

THE FREE RADICAL SCAVENGERS AND QUENCHERS

As discussed in Chapter 2, the single most important aspect of the protection of the body against radiation damage during and shortly after exposure is the deactivation of free radical activity. In this chapter, we explore evidence that such damage can be reduced by various specific *anti-oxidants,* and *free radical scavengers* or *quenchers,* acting to blot out the chain reaction of damage which these highly reactive particles can produce in DNA and cell membranes. As already discussed, it is this damage which can result in cancer, premature aging, and other abnormalities in cellular function.

Chapter 4 will consider those methods and substances potentially capable of enhancing the structural integrity of the cell membranes and reducing radiation effects in other, more general ways. Some of the nutrients, such as vitamin E, are involved in both free radical deactivation and cell membrane integrity, and so will be mentioned in both sections. We will then go on in Chapter 5 to specifically examine the issues and potential strategies involved in radiation therapy, applying many of the nutrients and principles introduced here.

The various protective nutrients will be discussed in this section in their "family" groups: vitamins, amino acids, enzymes, and minerals. The battle for survival in the presence of ionizing radiation is essentially a team effort, and it should be understood that the use of only one or another of these nutrients, with no regard to the rest, is as futile as a soccer team fielding its best striker and perhaps its goalkeeper, and not bothering about the rest of the team, or perhaps just sending in the reserves. On the other hand, not all protective approaches need to always be used simultaneously; there are often several ways to reach the same objective, and many factors can affect the approaches chosen. Increasingly, the traditional medical establishment and nutrition-ists are coming to agree with alternative practitioners on the efficacy of such nutritional support (see Machlin and Bendich, 1987).

VITAMINS

The vitamin family includes a number of powerful antioxidant protection agents. The three most important are vitamins A, C, and E. A number of others, including some of the B vitamins, also have a subsidiary role in free radical containment.

Vitamin A and Beta-Carotene

Vitamin A, a fat-soluble vitamin found in animal products, has strong antioxidant properties. Our bodies can also manufacture vitamin A from beta-carotene, which is obtained from plants. Beta-carotene is itself a very powerful antioxidant and is the form recommended most strongly for radiation protection, since it appears to be even more effective than vitamin A as an antioxidant and free-radical neutralizer, and it is almost totally nontoxic. This cannot be said for vitamin A itself, and caution is required with anything beyond mild supplementation. Excess vitamin A can cause unpleasant reactions, including vomiting, fatigue, headache, joint pain, skin reactions, and, in children, abnormal growth. (However, most symptoms of this sort disappear rapidly when normal intake is resumed, and long-term damage is almost unheard of unless the liver is already severely damaged.) Beta-carotene is preferable to vitamin A because it presents no such problems. The most that has been observed with excessive intake has been a mild diarrhea, which soon ceases spontaneously without the necessity for interruption of the beta-carotene supple-mentation. Much of the research to date has been done with vitamin A, but the results should also be applicable to its beta-carotene precursor.

The main function of vitamin A is to provide protection to mucous membranes, such as the epithelial linings of the intestinal tract and the lungs. It also plays important roles in tissue healing. In addition, cells that have become altered to forms considered precancerous are, with vitamin A's assistance, often capable of recovering and regaining normal function. This has been well discussed by Goodman, (1984). Furthermore, the more of the other antioxidant nutrients that are present in the body, such as vitamins C and E, the less vitamin A is required over and above the body's normal requirements for the provision of this protection. Vitamin A also has been shown to have strong protective capability against x-ray–induced damage, as is discussed in detail in Chapter 5.

Recent studies indicate that beta-carotene is an unusual antioxidant. Burton and Ingold (1984) showed that it has both an antioxidant capability and a role as a quencher of the reactive so-called "singlet oxygen," (the culprit in sunburn), and that its means of operation are quite novel. They concluded that beta-carotene plays an important role in protecting lipids from oxidative changes in the body; along with vitamin E, whose action it complements, it can break the chain of production of peroxyl radicals in much the same manner as the enzyme superoxide dismutase (SOD), which will be discussed.

Ames (1983) confirms that many of the harmful effects of ionizing radiation's damage to DNA and cells are due to generation of oxygen radicals and that beta-carotene is protective against this.

Of particular interest, beta-carotene is effective in tissues with low oxygen concentrations (such as tumors), in contrast to vitamin E, which operates best in tissues with high concentrations of oxygen, such as the outer lining of the lungs and the surface membranes of red blood cells. The implications of this fact are discussed further in Chapter 5.

Pizzorno and Murray (1986) discuss the evidence that the activity of beta-carotene in the human body is similar to its action in plants, where it functions as a cellular screen against light-induced oxidation and free-radical activity. Being fat soluble, it gets into the fatty membranes of cells and thus helps prevent peroxidation of the fatty acids, to maintain and protect the integrity of the cell structures.

Green and yellow plants are the main dietary source of beta-carotene. The darker the color, the greater the concentration of carotenoids, usually including beta-carotene. When beta-carotene is used as a supplement, it is recommended that it be taken in combination with substantial dietary sources of carotenoids. If adequate vitamin A is present in the diet from sources such as liver, kidney, butter, and whole milk, then the supplemental beta-carotene and other carotenoids will largely remain in the circulation unconverted and will be able to act in their antioxidant role. This would be of particular value in a program to minimize the effects of radiation (or any other source of free-radical activity).

**Suggested Dosage of Beta-Carotene:
25 to 40 milligrams daily**

Supplementation with vitamin A is not suggested unless specifically advised by a knowledgeable health professional, in which case a water-soluble form is advocated for ease of absorption.

Vitamin C

Vitamin C, or ascorbic acid, is a major antioxidant and defender of cell integrity. Most mammals make their own vitamin C, synthesizing a good deal more than normal in times of stress. Millions of years ago, primates and a few other mammals lost the genes for making vitamin C, presumably while living in lush forests with an abundance of green plants and fruits within easy reach to supply what thus became an essential vitamin. The needed vitamin C was near at hand, as it still is for the mountain gorilla. This loss only became a disadvantage when early humans, because of climatic upheavals, were obliged to seek and hunt other foods, in order to survive. Under the new conditions, with no way of switching the genetic machinery back to allow internal manufacture of vitamin C, we have to obtain through our now less perfect diet a sufficient daily intake of vitamin C, which, being water-soluble, cannot be stored. Though many dispute their claims, Pauling (1986), Cheraskin (1983), and many others argue quite forcefully that this often is not achieved in modern industrialized societies, particularly in times of stress and illness. They suggest that we need 500 to 2500 milligrams of vitamin C daily, even though official RDA levels are set at only 60–80 milligrams per day. There is substantial evidence pointing to a greater requirement, especially when the body is under stress, as it is during periods of radiation exposure.

Many nutrition textbooks and writers on health have suggested a wide variety of possible side-effects of doses of vitamin C in the gram range: kidney stones, vitamin B_{12} deficiency, infertility, rebound scurvy, and difficulty with certain diagnostic tests. The latter problem, while real, can be avoided by choice of test or reducing C intake immediately prior to the test. The other suggested complications are all based on very limited anecdotal information, which has not stood up to further scrutiny but somehow remains entrenched in the literature. For example, concern has been expressed about the possibility that high doses of vitamin C may produce kidney stones. However, all the textbook references to this danger seem to lead back to a single experiment with four subjects, one of whom got kidney stones (which may or may not have actually been related to the vitamin C). Were this actually a significant problem, one would expect far more extensive substantiation, considering the large numbers of people around the world using megadoses of the vitamin. Both Cathcart and Constance Tsao (1986) point to quite the opposite conclusion; their evidence suggests that the slight increase in acidity of the urine following high vitamin C intake, as well as increased subsequent urination, reduces the likelihood of oxalate kidney stones forming, even in those patients previously affected.

The indication of a potential B_{12} deficiency turned out to be due solely to flawed experimental technique; there is absolutely no evidence to support such a problem. Both Cheraskin (1983) and Pauling (1986) have excellent detailed analyses of the literature references supporting and refuting the various potential side-effects; in general, except in the case of individuals with a few rare genetic abnormalities, there is no substantiated evidence for significant side-effects even up to bowel tolerance levels.

Correlating intake of each of a wide variety of nutrients with general health status in a health professional population of over a thousand, Cheraskin and Ringsdorf (1977) have shown widespread vitamin C inadequacy in all strata of society in the United States. Basu and Schorah (1981) showed widespread evidence

of suboptimal vitamin C intake in the general population, and a
surprisingly high incidence of full-blown scurvy, the recognized
vitamin C deficiency disease, among elderly outpatients and
cancer patients, as well as in institutionalized young and old
people in the United States. They observed the following pattern:

Group	Suboptimal Vitamin C	Scurvy
Young healthy	3%	0%
Elderly healthy	20%	3%
Elderly outpatients	68%	20%
Cancer patients	76%	46%
Elderly institutionalized	95%	50%
Young institutionalized	100%	30%

Vitamin C is very important for radiation protection. It is a
significant part of the antiradiation mixture used in the Russian
space program. Animal studies have shown that vitamin C was
able to prevent the development of cancer on the skins of rodents
exposed to ultraviolet irradiation, apparently because of its powerful antioxidant qualities.

Cathcart (1985) reports administering *very* large amounts of
ascorbic acid in times of stress to achieve tissue saturation. He
suggests that the intake of vitamin C be increased by a gram daily
until bowel tolerance is reached. (This is the level of intake at
which diarrhea commences.) The ideal dosage is considered to
be that taken the day previously at which level of intake diarrhea
was not evident. This level of intake, which may reach 25–150
grams daily spread over four to six doses, is maintained until
normal health is regained. Diarrhea then commences, and the
dose is again reduced stepwise to stay within bowel tolerance. He
reports good results with burns, injury, and surgery, and in
conditions ranging from infections to allergies and more serious
degenerative diseases. Clearly, in this approach ascorbic acid is
being used pharmacologically and not nutritionally at such
levels, although, as Cathcart points out, the patient who can
tolerate without diarrhea an intake of 15 grams daily of vitamin C
when well, will be able to tolerate 10–15 times that amount when
seriously ill (with viral pneumonia, for example).

The high levels of intake just discussed are suggested for use
only under the guidance of a qualified health professional. These
guidelines might be employed when substantial radiation expo-

sure is current or likely. It should be noted that some concern has been expressed on the basis of animal studies, that dehydroascorbic acid, formed during oxidation from ascorbic acid (vitamin C), might itself cause tissue damage. Cathcart has considered this, and maintains that there are substantial differences between the two situations and that, in humans, the likelihood of such toxicity is small. This issue appears unresolved. Thus, it is suggested that use of high intakes of vitamin C be stopped prior, for example, to radiotherapy, to be recommenced as soon after therapy as possible, unless further data are obtained and/or specific advice to the contrary is given by a qualified health professional.

Suggested dosage of Vitamin C:
0.5 to 3 grams daily, possibly with elevation to
bowel tolerance under certain circumstances

Vitamin E

Vitamin E is also a fat-soluble vitamin whose major (if not only) role is to act as a free-radical deactivator and antioxidant. Vitamin E is a major protector of lipids in cell membranes and has been shown to protect DNA from damage and mutation when exposed to radiation (cf. Beckman et al., 1982; Cook and McNamara, (1980).

Several studies, reviewed by Sarria and Prasad (1984, their references 1–8) have shown that vitamin E protects normal tissues of the body against radiation damage. Those authors also discuss evidence that vitamin E does not protect tumor cells but may actually enhance the effect of radiation on those tissues; in Chapter 5, we explore further the exciting possibility that supplementation of vitamin E in radiotherapy both protects the healthy tissues and makes the tumor cells more vulnerable.

As discussed by Borek et al. (1986), vitamin E and the mineral selenium have a synergistic relationship in which they enhance each other's beneficial protective effects against free-radical activity and radiation damage to cells, each acting via a different mechanism. However, supplemental vitamin E should not be used by patients with cancer of the breast, since there is some evidence that it has a hormone-like activity that can enhance growth of that particular kind of tumor.

**Suggested dosage of
Vitamin E (d-alpha-tocopherol):
400 to 800 international units daily;
this should be in a water-soluble form
for ease of absorption**

The B Vitamins

Several nutrients that have central roles in the main processes of
metabolism of amino acids, fatty acids, and sugars are grouped
into the B complex. Some of them are vitally involved in antiradiation activity, although they themselves have little or no
direct antioxidant activity. Some supplementation may well be
helpful—preferably in divided doses to maintain serum levels—but there are no data on which to suggest specific doses.
One should probably not go above 10 times the RDA without
specific indication.

Vitamin B₁ (Thiamine). This water-soluble nutrient is essential
to the processes that produce energy in the body, as well as to
most other aspects of metabolism. Along with vitamin C and the
sulfur-containing amino acid cysteine, of which we will hear more
later, it appears to also help protect the tissues against cross-
linkage damage to protein.

Vitamins B₂ (Riboflavin) and B₃ (Niacinamide). These vitamins
have a supporting role as antioxidants with free-radical scaveng-
ing activity.

Vitamin B₅ (Pantothenic Acid). This vitamin, which is often
available as calcium pantothenate, is important to the function of
the adrenal gland and plays many roles in the body relating to
stress-induced damage, especially of the neural structures. Pantothenic acid reportedly reduces cross-linkage damage in the
tissues and enhances the functioning of the immune system. Its
major direct function is as a component of a molecule (acetyl
CoA) that has a central role in metabolism of carbohydrates, fat,
and proteins. No definite RDA has yet been established; Japanese researchers have some evidence that it may be five times
the 4–7 milligrams per day listed as the "reasonable and safe"
levels.

Animal studies in Hungary (Szorady, 1963) showed that when mice were given pantothenic acid supplementally and were then exposed to high doses of radiation, their survival rates were twice that of control mice, which received no supplementation.

Suggested dosage of Pantothenic Acid:
25 to 100 milligrams daily
in divided doses

Vitamin B₆ (Pyridoxine). This is a most important nutrient, as it is a constituent part of numerous enzymes and is involved in producing several hormones, playing a major role in immune function. Adequate amounts of vitamin B_6 are particularly necessary for amino acid metabolism.

Many radiologists have found that giving patients supplementary vitamin B_6 helps allay the symptoms of nausea which may accompany radiotherapy.

Levels may be depleted because of oral contraceptives, smoking, or alcohol consumption. Neurotoxicity of vitamin B_6 is possible with very high doses, more than approximately 400 milligrams per day. In many of its functions, vitamin B_6 interacts with zinc, another nutrient that will be discussed.

Suggested dosage of B_6:
50 milligrams three times daily
in divided doses

Brewers' yeast: another method of obtaining the B vitamins is by taking brewers' yeast in tablet or powder form in large amounts, about 3 tablespoons of powder or 12 tablets daily. However, caution is required in taking brewers' yeast in case of extensive *Candida albicans* infection or if there is an allergy or sensitivity to yeast. If *Candida albicans* is a problem, such symptoms as bloatedness, nausea, dizziness, and fatigue are often noted when yeast-based foods are eaten. Chaitow's book *Candida Albicans: Could Yeast Be Your Problem?* (Thorsons, 1985) may be of some help. Yeast is actually the source of most B-vitamin supplements, but yeast-free sources are available.

Bioflavonoids. This group of nutrient substances, while not shown to be essential vitamins, are known to assist in many important functions, not least in aiding the ability of vitamin C to perform its antioxidant and tissue-repair activities (cf. J. Bland, 1984).

The bioflavonoids are found in large amounts in the rinds of citrus fruits and in many other fruits and herbs. Like vitamin C, they enhance immune system function, and together they have powerful anti-inflammatory capabilities (Pizzorno and Murray, 1986). Among their many other areas of usefulness is an anti-radiation protection role. Some, such as rutin, the flavonoid extracted from buckwheat, have the ability to help increase the strength of capillary walls. Quercitin is another flavonoid, extracted from a tree bark, and has powerful anti-inflammatory and cell-protective abilities. Many of the bioflavonoids are part of the Russian antiradiation formulation provided to cosmonauts (Saksonov, 1975).

Dosage suggestion for Bioflavonoids:
1 to 2 grams daily with Vitamin C

ENZYME ANTIOXIDANTS AND TRACE MINERALS

We have many enzyme systems available to help protect against oxidants and free radicals. The most important are catalase and superoxide dismutase.

One major substance involved in the defense of the body against free-radical activity is the powerful enzyme superoxide dismutase (SOD). Unsuccessful attempts have been made to boost SOD activity (or that of other intracellular enzymes) via supplementation. While SOD in the body is indeed one of the best protectors against damage triggered by radiation (or by other factors such as heavy-metal toxicity), taking SOD by mouth does not raise its level in the body because it is too large to pass through the wall of the digestive tract or to get from there into individual cells. However, to produce active SOD the body needs the minerals copper, manganese, and zinc, and supplementation of these does indeed have the ability to enhance SOD production.

A recent report in *The New Scientist* indicates that medical science is moving towards a greater understanding of this potential enhancement of SOD activity through supplementation. Scientists at the University of Arkansas have synthesized copper derivatives that can induce protection against radiation damage via enhancement of SOD activity. Mice given this copper were sufficiently protected to allow almost 60% of them to survive what is considered to be a lethal radiation dose. Moderate supplemental dosages of copper, zinc, and manganese therefore appear desirable in the promotion of SOD protection for cells challenged by radiation. (Zinc is also especially crucial in various other aspects of cell and tissue healing, as will be discussed further in the next chapter.)

Two other recent developments hold potential promise for the long term. Bland (1984) suggests that *copper salicylate* has superoxide-scavenging properties like those of SOD, which make it a very effective protective agent against tumor development. Copper salicylates also have an important function in maintaining the levels of glutathione in the liver, which, as will be described, is a very important part of the antioxidant system preventing free-radical damage. However, copper salicylates are not yet generally available, so one generally must rely on other sources of copper.

To enhance SOD production
the following nutrients are recommended:

Zinc	**15 to 30 milligrams daily**
Manganese	**5 to 20 milligrams daily**
Copper	**1 to 5 milligrams daily**
	(as salicylate, if available)

Copper and zinc compete for absorption, and excessive copper is toxic. Taking the two in a ratio of 1:10 to 1:20 seems to give a reasonable balance of both. Another approach used in Europe is a rotation system in which zinc is taken for 5 days a week and copper for 2. However, this seems less desirable in terms of maintaining optimal tissue levels.

These nutrients should be taken with meals and should be used as supplements for a time beyond any period of exposure to radiation.

The enzyme *glutathione peroxidase*, which contains the mineral selenium, helps glutathione—a molecule made of three amino acids—to inactivate hydrogen peroxide inside cells. Thus, poor functioning of this enzyme reduces the efficiency with which free radicals are contained and prevented from damaging tissues (Meister, 1983).

Direct supplementation with glutathione peroxidase is impossible (as with SOD), but there is strong evidence that supplementation with selenium is effective in protecting from free-radical damage; in fact, acting as a cofactor for this enzyme is the major role of selenium. This evidence is discussed further in Chapter 5, on radiation therapy. However, Meister points out that during chemotherapy treatment of cancer, such supplementation might actually diminish the effectiveness of the drugs by amplifying the action of glutathione peroxidase, which detoxifies some of these drugs in the tissues, thus reducing their cancer-destroying actions. Anyone undergoing simultaneous radiotherapy and chemotherapy should therefore consult the physician prior to supplementation with selenium. In protecting against radiation damage, one might be reducing the effectiveness of the chemotherapy.

Several animal studies conducted in Europe have reported on the protective effect of selenium against radiation that would normally have proved fatal (Colombetti, 1969; Badiello, 1970). Borek and his colleagues, at Columbia University College of Physicians and Surgeons (1986), reported on a study in which both selenium and vitamin E were given as supplements to cultured mouse embryo prior to irradiation. Cells receiving selenium contained more glutathione peroxidase and glutathione, and consequently they had enhanced abilities to destroy peroxide and thus survive radiation. The combination of vitamin E and selenium enhanced the protective effect. Vitamin E acting alone protected against x-rays and other toxic factors, but not against peroxide. The research team concluded that "initiation of the neoplastic process [development of cancer cells] induced by radiation (or chemicals) can be prevented by nontoxic levels of selenium and vitamin E." They believe that the anticarcinogenic actions of selenium and vitamin E are achieved by different mechanisms but that they act in concert, underscoring the concept that "appropriate measures in our lifestyle can lower the rate of human affliction to cancer."

To enhance
glutathione peroxidase production
the following nutrient is suggested:
Selenium   400 micrograms daily

AMINO ACIDS

Amino acids are the building blocks of protein. Our bodies require 20 of them to construct the enzymes and other proteins that constitute such an important part of our structure. We normally obtain them by breaking down the long-chain protein molecules in our food into short fragments or individual amino acids, using digestive enzymes in the acid environment of the gut. Twelve of the amino acids can, in adult life, also be produced within the body from other amino acids. The other eight, however, have to be present in our food all at the same time in sufficient quantity to support needed protein synthesis; otherwise, we have to break down muscle, blood, and liver proteins to obtain them.

Many important roles have been discovered for several of the amino acids in addition to their main function as the constituents of protein, and some are being used to great advantage in treating ill health, as discussed in detail by Chaitow (1985). Since they are part of the normal economy of the body, they tend to be handled more safely than synthetic drugs. In general, however, they should not be used indiscriminately; there can be harmful results from their misuse. (For example, phenylalanine, a major constituent of Nutrasweet, can lead to brain damage in people with genetic defects in metabolizing it. The extreme form of such a defect is phenylketonuria.) At higher doses they function pharmacologically, not as nutrients, and the potential for harmful imbalances exists, particularly for those that become neurotransmitters. This potential appears to be low, however, with the amino acids other than tryptophan suggested here, particularly when they are not taken at meals.

Glutathione

The major amino-acid support suggested against free radicals is from the triple amino-acid compound glutathione, which we noted as being the major factor in the protective activity of the enzyme glutathione peroxidase. Glutathione is a powerful antioxidant, acting outside cells as well as in them, and its effectiveness is greatly enhanced by glutathione peroxidase inside cells acting to restore it to its active state.

Glutathione is made up of three amino acids: cysteine, glutamine, and glycine. Its many protective roles include anticancer properties, heavy metal detoxification, slowing of the aging process, and enhanced liver detoxification of environmental pollutants, drugs, and alcohol. Glutathione also enhances the antioxidant effects of vitamin C.

The evidence indicates that glutathione, while taken up intact from the gut, is only poorly taken into most cells unless it is in an altered chemical form (such as an ethyl ester). Instead, it is degraded on the cell surface. However, supplemental glutathione still shows a definite protective effect, perhaps by supplying cells simultaneously with the particular three amino acids needed to make new glutathione. In fact, glutathione is normally made primarily in the liver and shipped from there to all parts of the body as a way of supplying other cells with its important component amino acids, particularly during starvation. It thus appears to be particularly important to supplement with glutathione when the liver is functioning poorly. Taking cysteine directly is not as effective in enhancing cellular glutathione levels.

However, Meister et al. (1986) also argues that the presence of glutathione during radiation therapy may reduce the effectiveness of the radiation in killing certain kinds of cancer cells, particularly some that are normally radiation resistant. It is possible that depletion of glutathione makes cells more susceptible to irradiation. This factor ought to be taken into account when glutathione and cysteine supplementation prior to a course of radiotherapy is considered, particularly if the radiation is very tightly directed on the tumor area so that relatively little healthy tissue is affected. On the other hand, anyone exposed to diagnostic radiation (or any other source) could safely use the dosages given here:

**Dosage of glutathione should be
between 1 and 3 grams daily,
during periods of radiation exposure,
but not during radiation therapy.
Use divided doses away from meal times.**

Cysteine

One of the components of glutathione is the sulfur-containing amino acid cysteine. This is itself a powerful antioxidant and detoxification agent and is capable of deactivating free radicals. When combined with vitamin C and vitamin B_1, cysteine has a protective effect on cells exposed to radiation. There is a caution for diabetics, who should not take cysteine supplementally without guidance, as it is capable of reducing certain disulfide bonds in insulin (cf. Pearson and Shaw, 1983).

Cysteine should be taken together with vitamin C, in a dosage of three times the intake of cysteine to enhance its protective effect, and with vitamin B_6 (50 milligrams of B_6, in the form of pyridoxal-5phosphate) per gram of cysteine (Philpott, 1983). Its use is suggested when there is exposure to radiation, especially if glutathione is unavailable or undesirable.

**Dosage of cysteine recommended is
1 to 3 grams daily
to accompany glutathione or instead of
glutathione, during periods of radiation exposure.
Take cysteine away from meal times in divided
doses with water or a juice.**

The much-publicized Russian antiradiation mixture mentioned earlier includes vitamins C, B_1, B_6, and bioflavonoids; the amino acids histidine and tryptophan; and the trace elements zinc and selenium, as well as the adaptogen ginseng (Saksonov, 1975; Brekhman, 1980). Most of these substances will be discussed in the following pages, but at this point the two amino acids in the mixture, histidine and tryptophan, deserve attention.

Histidine

Histidine has been used effectively in the treatment of rheumatoid arthritis (Pfeiffer, 1975). It is thought to have its desirable effects via its ability to tightly bind, or *chelate*, heavy metals and aid in their removal from the system. This, however, does not account for its value in radiation exposure, unless it reflects an inhibition of some hitherto unreported (though not unlikely) synergistic effect between heavy metals and radiation in inducing oxidation. It may also increase the absorption of trace minerals.

Histidine is also reported to be necessary for the maintenance of the myelin sheath, which protects and insulates nerve structures (Bormann, 1975). This is one place where antiradiation protection might be achieved, for in the first overwhelming wave of radiation the nervous system is one of the most vulnerable. It is therefore best to think of histidine as offering protection rather than being of value after radiation exposure. Russian cosmonauts take their protective mixture some 15 minutes prior to anticipated exposure, and this could be a useful strategy for those receiving radiotherapy.

**Suggested dosage of histidine:
1 to 2 grams daily;
as with all amino acids, this should be taken away
from mealtimes with water or juice.**

Caution: Certain forms of manic depressive illness are characterized by the presence of excessive amounts of histamine, which derives from histidine, and individuals with such problems should probably avoid histidine supplementation.

Tryptophan

Tryptophan is an amino acid with no obvious antiradiation capability. However, it is used to make the neurotransmitter serotonin, and functions as an antidepressant and to enhance relaxation and sleep (especially when taken with vitamin B_6 and magnesium). Its value in the Russian nutrient cocktail could well lie in its stress-reducing abilities rather than in any ability to protect against radiation directly.

In summary, it is clear that at least glutathione and cysteine are potentially of importance in any program attempting to limit the damage that would result from radiation exposure.

RNA AND URIC ACID

Ribonucleic acid, or RNA, has been touted as a radiation-protective agent by several groups, particularly in Germany. There does seem to be evidence that it can be effective in enhancing the destruction of free radicals. Ames et al. (1981) have shown that plasma uric acid—the major RNA breakdown product—is one of the major systemic antioxidants in humans.

It is a powerful scavenger of free radicals and singlet oxygen, protecting effectively against membrane peroxidation and lysis in the test tube in laboratory experiments. It is about as effective an antioxidant as vitamin C and is present at much higher concentration in blood plasma (about 300 micromolar, compared with 30–85 micromolar for C). The levels naturally increase in response to oxidative stress – such as lead exposure, high alcohol ingestion, heavy exercise, and obesity – possibly as a way of coping with the higher concentrations of oxygen, with its reactive potential for damage. (As with vitamin C, however, there has been some suggestion that the oxidized urea may itself be able to cause some membrane damage, indicating reason for some caution in raising levels indiscriminately.

Eating uric acid directly has no effect on plasma levels, but eating yeast RNA can increase human levels at a rate of about 1 milligram per 100 milliliters of serum for each gram of RNA eaten, up to a level of 8 grams of RNA per day. This approach would of course be strongly counterindicated for anyone predisposed to gout, which is a physiological reaction to high uric acid levels.

Some researchers have suggested that there might be an organ-specific RNA protective effect, by which the RNA is actually able to still function as a messenger to direct protein synthesis under conditions in which the cell's own information has been damaged. In light of our current understanding of molecular and cellular biology, however, this mechanism is not possible. Cells do not take up RNA intact; if they did, that would allow foreign influences to alter or destroy crucial regulatory functions within the cell. Furthermore, there are very potent "ribonuclease" enzymes everywhere in nature – even on your own hands –-that rapidly and effectively break up the long RNA molecules, so that the specific informational messages in mRNA are rapidly destroyed. Also, there is no mechanism for the cell to recognize its own species of RNA, and any possible such effect would be extremely short-lived and of little help to a cell whose information is so badly damaged that it needs that assistance.

However, evidence for the nonspecific effect of RNA as an antioxidant comes from a number of studies. A report in *Radiation Research* (Sugahara et al., 1966) showed that animals which had been exposed to x-irradiation survived longer when injected at the same time with a preparation of yeast RNA, three times weekly. In 1960, Maisen and colleagues demonstrated that it was possible to increase rat survival rates from 4–5% to 60–65% via injection of RNA. Other researchers showed this to also be true in guinea pigs (Wagner and Silverman, 1984).

Dosage of RNA:
1–4 grams daily, in divided doses.

CHAPTER FOUR

MORE GENERAL PROTECTION AND REGENERATION OF BODY TISSUES

Our major focus in the last two chapters has been on directly reducing the production of radiation damage by making use of free radical quenchers and scavengers. That approach is mainly of use immediately during and after the actual time of radiation exposure. We now move on to explore ways, many of them less well understood, which may help prevent and repair damage to cell structures such as membranes and may more generally enhance cell healing. (It should be noted that some of the antioxidants and free radical scavengers already discussed also have this sort of broader effect.) Here, we will look at specific nutrients such as essential fatty acids, zinc, and the accessory nutrients inositol and choline, as well as at so-called *adaptogens* such as ginseng, eleutherococcus, and pollen.

ZINC

Zinc is a trace mineral which is essential to the activity of about 100 enzymes, including many of those involved in cellular protection and repair processes: DNA polymerase, RNA polymerase, thymidylate synthetase, alcohol dehydrogenase, one form of superoxide dismutase. The supplies in our diet often seem to be borderline, and deficiencies can develop very rapidly. For example, Hurley and Shrader (1975) have shown that when rats are on a normal diet until impregnated and then put on a zinc-free diet, abnormalities in the fetus can develop by the second or third day — by the four-cell stage — while the embryo is still in the fallopian tube, long before the placenta develops. Human studies by several authors have shown that when humans are receiving a zinc-depleted diet, serum levels can drop by a factor of at least 2 within a few weeks. Alcoholics in particular are often deficient. Lead, cesium, and copper also compete with zinc. To date, little research seems to have been directed at the potential usefulness of zinc in radiation protection, unfortunately. We have been only aware of the extent of its general importance in the body since the 1970s. However, a good deal of research has firmly established its role in supporting wound healing, the immune system, fetal development, and general tissue integrity as well as in superoxide dismutase. Thus, it seems appropriate to emphasize the importance of adequate zinc nutrition, particularly during times of stress and need for tissue repair, such as during exposure to radiation. Zinc is present in most high-protein foods, which are also important during periods of tissue repair. Supplementing with 15 to 25 milligrams per day of zinc may also well be appropriate. Almost any zinc salt can reasonably be used, but research indicates that zinc picolinate is taken up most efficiently (cf. Barrie et al., 1987).

ESSENTIAL FATTY ACIDS

The lipid components of the cell membranes are particularly vulnerable to lipid peroxidation and other forms of free-radical damage, as discussed in Chapter 2. These membranes are continually undergoing repair, slipping in new cholesterol and fatty acids and carting off old ones packaged in low-density lipoproteins to be processed by the liver.

Most membrane components can be made in our bodies; however, there are a few we cannot make. These are the most highly unsaturated ones, i.e., the fatty acids containing the most double bonds, such as *linoleic acid,* which are thus the most susceptible to damage. They are thus essential nutrients, termed *essential fatty acids,* or EFAs. In addition to their role in membrane structure, they have crucial regulatory functions. They routinely are clipped out of the membranes to be transformed into some of the most important messenger molecules carrying signals between nearby cells: the prostaglandins, thromboxanes, and leukotrienes, which are particularly important in the functioning of the immune system.

The range of biological activities of the prostaglandins is staggering. They are a complex family, found in nearly every tissue of the body. Minute amounts affect nearly every biological process, with at least one prostaglandin being inhibitory and another excitatory in most instances, so that important delicate balances must be maintained. One indication of the widespread impact and importance of this group of molecules is the fact that the only direct effect of *aspirin* is to inhibit the production of prostaglandins; they are thus involved in fever induction, inflammation, and pain. Cortisone also seems to act through prostaglandin-dependent mechanisms, and one group of prostaglandins are powerful agents for inducing labor.

There are two groups of essential fatty acids. The best studied is the so-called *"ω6" (omega-6) fatty acid* family (called this because their last double bond is exactly six carbons from the end of the fatty acid chain). This includes *linoleic acid* and two derivatives, which are the direct precursors of the two major classes of prostaglandins: *gamma-linolenic acid* and *arachidonic acid*. All members of this group can be interconverted in our bodies. They are found in seeds (including sunflower, sesame, and pumpkin seeds) and such oils as safflower, sunflower, linseed, and also evening primrose oil, a particularly rich source of the gamma linolenic form, which is sometimes specifically used in the attempt to affect the balance between prostaglandin classes.

The other essential fatty acid group, found only in fish and plankton from cold ocean waters, includes *alpha-linolenic acid, eicosapentaneoic acid (EPA)* and their derivatives. These so-called *"ω3" (omega-3) fatty acids,* which have double bonds to within three carbons from the end of the chain, are not interconvertible with the omega-6 group. They are used to make the third family of prostaglandins, whose role is not yet well understood. In some ways, ω3 fatty acids compete with the omega-6 group, and this has been considered potentially problematic; yet, recent research around the country has indicated substantial health

health advantages, particularly with regard to cardiovascular disease, for people on diets high in EPA from cold-water ocean fish. Inclusion of EPA into their diet is thus strongly encouraged.

This general understanding of the roles of essential fatty acids is relatively recent, and there still seems to be little research directly aimed at examining potential effects in radiation protection, so our suggestions can be based only on general knowledge and evidence carried over from other areas. We know that such highly unsaturated fats are very susceptible to free-radical oxidation damage, and that they can themselves be converted into very reactive oxidation products in the process; this is what is going on when oils turn rancid, and is partially prevented when vitamin E is added to the oil as a stabilizer.

The most prudent course of action seems to be to pay particular attention to eating a variety of very fresh good dietary sources of essential fatty acids during the days and months following radiation exposure, when membrane repair is particularly crucial. This should include a variety of seeds; fresh, cold-pressed oils; and such fish as salmon, mackerel, and herring. After but not during the exposure some supplementation with EFAs of various kinds, such as linseed oil and the fish extract maxEPA might be considered, probably at a level of four to six 500-milligram capsules a day, in an attempt to optimize the amount available for repair of crucial membrane functions.

ACCESSORY NUTRIENTS

The roles of vitamins, minerals, and essential fatty acids in human nutrition have been established through years of clinical and biochemical research. Their crucial functions in activating specific enzymes and serving as cellular communication signals and protective agents are now accepted. As has been discussed, their therapeutic usefulness when given in doses above that of the Recommended Daily Allowances is receiving increasing attention.

Another class of nutrients concentrated from food is now also receiving significant attention: the *accessory nutrients*.

There has been some confusion and controversy in the nutrition literature about these substances. They are not "essential nutrients" in the sense that they can be made in our bodies at levels which would be considered "adequate" for most individuals; including them with the B vitamins is thus often severely criticized. However, there are increasing indications that they may not be made at optimum levels for the promotion of health, at least under certain circumstances; so there may be justification for providing them through supplementation or paying attention to dietary sources under some circumstances even though they are not "vitamins" in the traditional sense. Using the name "accessory nutrients" helps make this distinction clearer.

The general role of accessory nutrients may be better understood by looking at such essential nutrients as vitamins B_3 and D. These are called vitamins even though they can be produced to some degree in the human body and thus fall outside the normal rigorous definition of vitamins. For example, vitamin B_3 (niacin) can be manufactured in the liver from dietary tryptophan, although not at levels adequate to meet the needs even of most healthy people. Thus, pellagra results if niacin is not also supplied in adequate amounts in the diet. Similarly, vitamin D can be produced in the skin by exposure to full-spectrum sunlight, but the prevalence of rickets when dietary vitamin D is low attests to the general inadequacy of this source. Accessory nutrients, as mentioned, also seem to not be made at optimum levels in our bodies. Until and unless a frank deficiency disease is associated with dietary lack of any of the accessory nutrients, they are not appropriately called vitamins; this is a point made strongly by most nutrition books. There does seem to be growing evidence, however, that they may still be very useful in improving health under some circumstances. Bland (1982) has produced a very good, readable discussion of these accessory nutrients and many of their roles.

Inositol and Choline

The accessory nutrients *choline* and *inositol* both are crucial parts of membrane phospholipids as phosphatidylcholine and the phosphatidylinositol family, respectively. Both have important functions in addition to their direct role as membrane lipids. Phosphatidylcholine acts as a reservoir of choline with which nerve cells can synthesize the neurotransmitter *acetylcholine.* Acetylcholine is essential at the junction between nerves and muscles and in the parasympathetic nervous system, controlling many homeostatic mechanisms throughout the body, as well as playing many essential roles in the brain.

Phosphatidylinositol 4, 5-bisphosphate, one of the membrane lipids, also has recently been shown to play a crucial role in cell–cell communication. It is needed to translate signals brought to the cell surface by many kinds of hormones into intracellular messages and effects. The mechanism, though very complex, is worth looking at briefly, for a sense of the complexity of the roles and interactions in membranes and the importance of precise structures to their proper functioning.

Binding of a hormone, such as acetylcholine, to receptors on cells of the exocrine pancreas or smooth muscle triggers an enzyme to cut the phosphatidylinositol 4,5-bisphosphate into two pieces. One of these activates another enzyme, called a "protein kinase," that changes the rate of activity of all sorts of enzymes in the cell and is involved in regulating cell division. The other triggers release of calcium from stores inside the cell and thus precipitates such responses as contraction of the muscle. (For an excellent if rather technical review, see Agranoff, 1986, and the succeeding group of papers from the 1985 American Society for Pharmacology meeting, appearing in the same journal issue.)

In view of the crucial roles of these "second messengers," it appears particularly important to have ample stores of inositol and choline at times of membrane damage and extensive repair, although there are not yet many direct data dealing with their effects during radiation exposure. Adequate sources appear to be particularly crucial in protecting the fetus and infant, since both nutrients are essential to myelin sheath formation. (Supplementation with choline sources also gives marked improvement with certain neurological problems, such as Alzheimer's disease, but there does not seem to be good evidence that it generally enhances memory, as is sometimes claimed.)

There is substantial evidence that supplementation can affect serum levels positively for these nutrients (cf. Bland, 1982). Choline is even able to get across the blood–brain barrier—which most substances cannot cross—and substantially affects levels in the cerebrospinal fluid. There is substantial evidence that using phosphatidylcholine—one of several components of lecithin—works much better and with fewer side problems than does choline itself. Unfortunately, most lecithin available at health food stores contains only a very small amount of the choline derivatives; for therapeutic purposes, it is crucial that they make up at least one third of the lecithin.

Suggested Dose:
10 to 20 grams daily of
phosphatidylcholine-enriched lecithin

PABA

Para-aminobenzoic acid (PABA) also falls into this group. One of its major uses is in sun creams, to cut down potentially carcinogenic ultraviolet damage to the skin, and it may also be useful in protecting cell membranes, but there is little evidence on this subject. PABA, choline, and lecithin are frequently included in B-vitamin tablets, partly because they are already found in the yeast or other sources from which the B vitamins are being made.

ADAPTOGENS

An adaptogen is a substance which nonspecifically helps the body to adapt to stress without harmful side-effects. To qualify as an adaptogen, the substance should have protective properties of a general nature, thus enhancing a wide range of functions and protecting against a wide variety of potentially harmful factors. In saying that its effects should be *nonspecific*, we mean that an adaptogen should be able to enhance the body's own recuperative powers, homeostasis, and balancing and normalizing functions, whatever the nature of the problem, in contrast to such substances as painkillers or tranquilizers, which have specific pharmaceutical effects. Adaptogens should thus be useful in protecting against the damaging effects of radiation, whatever these might involve. The best-studied adaptogens are ginseng, eleutherococcus, royal jelly, and pollen.

Ginseng

Ginseng is an adaptogen that has been used in the Orient for thousands of years as a substance which prolongs the active period of life. A series of four proceedings of the International Ginseng Symposium, published by the Korean Ginseng and Tobacco Institute, extensively document the biochemical properties and physiological effects of various forms of ginseng (Park et al, 1974, 1978, 1980, 1984). Specifically regarding radiation damage, Japanese studies (Takeda et al., 1981) have shown a strong protective role for ginseng. Mice were injected with a

partially purified ginseng extract before or after receiving whole
body radiation. It was found that the effectiveness of the ginseng
did not vary with mode of injection, either into the peritoneum or
intravenously. The study used four groups of 40 mice and varied
injection from 2 days prior to radiation exposure to 2.5 hours
afterwards (using 720 rad). The efficacy of the protection was
judged by a variety of measurements. Ginseng was most effective
if given either 1 or 2 days prior to radiation exposure but was
found ineffective if given 3 days or more beforehand. Treatment
1 day after was also not effective but when received just hours
afterwards still offered significant protection: there was a decrease in spleen weight of irradiated mice to about one third of
normal, with those receiving ginseng regaining normal weight by
10 days after exposure, while those receiving a placebo injection
of saline (salt water) took 30 days to recover spleen weight, if
they survived. Fully 75% of the high-dosage ginseng rats survived for 30 days as against 14% of the placebo group. A variety
of blood level determinations showed similar results.

This clearly seems to fit the pattern of nonspecific protective
effects characteristic of adaptogens—the ability to adapt to the
stresses and toxicities of radiation, in this instance. Adaptogens
have not as yet yielded up the secrets of their active constituents,
but a good deal of effort is being expended in this direction, as is
evidenced by subsequent papers by the authors of this study that
examine the effects of various ginseng extracts under similar
conditions. Further research has been published in the Ginseng
Symposia. For example, Park et al. (1984) have characterized a
strong antioxidant in ginseng. In this regard, red Korean ginseng
was found to have twice the activity of white ginseng.

Eleutherococcus

Eleutherococcus is a Siberian plant which has properties similar
to ginseng. It reportedly raised the lifespan of rats by 16.5% and
is known to be a powerful antioxidant, so it also fits with the
nutrients discussed in the last chapter. It enhances endurance
and, as would be anticipated from an adaptogen, it reduces the
effect of all types of stress, with no reported side-effects.

Russian scientists investigating antiradiation methods give
prime place to these two adaptogens, ginseng, and eleutherococcus, since they were found to increase resistance more pro-
foundly and to a wider range of unfavorable effects, whether
chemical, physical, or biological, than any other substance stud-

ied. For example, Brekhman (1980) tells of Russian experiments in which mice were subjected to highly toxic substances and in which high doses of ginseng and eleutherococcus were able to offer a substantial degree of protection.

Royal Jelly

Royal jelly, secreted by worker bees to feed their queen, also has the characteristics of an adaptogen. It is extremely rich in a wide range of nutrients and is, for example, one of the best sources of pantothenic acid (vitamin B_5), found by Roger Williams, its discoverer, to increase lifespan 15% in experimental animals and retard general deterioration (cf. Williams, 1979). Bulgarian researchers (Peichev, 1966) report that royal jelly has an ability to protect against radiation, as well as to generally reduce the effects of stress.

Pollen

Pollen is another nonspecific nutrient source which has also been reported to have a protective effect in both cancer patients and animals receiving radiation, as discussed in the next chapter.

There is no way at present of knowing whether these effects relate to the presence of nutrients, such as those discussed in the previous chapter, which may be present in these adaptogens, or whether there are other as yet unidentified substances acting in a protective manner. Essential fatty acids are, for example, plentiful in pollen. The effectiveness of adaptogens may well reflect a good balance of a wide variety of substances rather than any particular small group of nutrients.

With any adaptogen it is necessary to take the substance regularly and for some time before a noticeable effect is produced. A gram or two a day of ginseng or eleutherococcus is suggested, and a month or more should be anticipated before benefits are felt. With radiation damage, this is a long time to wait, so the regular use of such substances in everyday life as nonspecific protective agents is indicated for those who risk exposure to radiation and other free radicals. Regular use might very possibly have a positive effect on general health as well.

All in all, the various nutrients discussed here seem to have strong potential for helping to maintain and regain general health in times of severe stress, including that imposed by exposure to ionizing radiation.

CHAPTER FIVE

RADIOTHERAPY:
Enhancing Its Benefits and Reducing Its Dangers

Radiotherapy presents a unique set of challenges. In it, the attempt is made to selectively kill off certain cells (the cancer) without damaging healthy body cells too seriously. The problem is represented in Figure 7.

We will discuss here nutritional approaches aimed at broadening the distance between these two curves, termed "improving the therapeutic ratio," by enhancing tumor killing and/or by protecting the cells in the rest of the body. Fractionating the dose into several smaller treatments separated by set periods of time also is used to help accomplish this purpose. The careful choice of doses is crucial to enhancing therapeutic effects. The therapeutic ratio is also affected by recent technical advances such as improved focusing of the radiation beam on the tumor and, for some purposes, the use of beams of neutrons rather than x-rays or gamma rays. The best nutritional approach may well be affected by the kind and format of radiation being used as well as the nature of the cancer. In addition, it must be borne in mind that the radiation itself may have profound effects on the nutritional status, particularly the ability to take up nutrients, if the head, neck, abdomen, or pelvis is irradiated. Such patients normally lose at least 10% of their body weight during a 6–8 week course of therapy.

Figure 7.
Relationship between radiation dose,
lethality to cancer cells, and damage to
healthy body tissue.

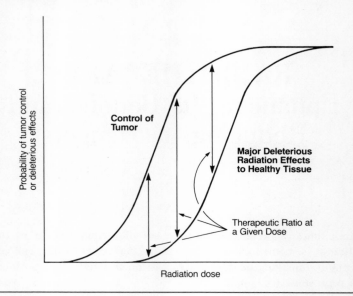

Patients' responses to radiotherapy are highly variable. They
depend upon such factors as the stage of the disease and the site
being treated, as well as the precise protocol and such elements,
often intangible, as the overall prior nutritional status of the
patient. As discussed in the *Cancer Manual* of the Massachusetts
Division of the American Cancer Society (1982), at least four
important biological parameters can be influenced by *dose fractionation*, which affects the therapeutic ratio. It appears very
likely that these same factors may well be affected further by
close attention to nutritional parameters during treatment. They
are as follows:

1. Repair of sublethal radiation damage to membranes,
DNA, and other vital structures in both normal and tumor cells;
the first is clearly advantageous to the patient, the second detri-
mental to treatment.

2. Division of surviving tumor cells, repopulating the tumor.

3. Reassortment of surviving normal and tumor cells into other phases of the cell cycle. (This is important, since cells are primarily susceptible to radiation during the phase when DNA is replicating, so a new group of cells may become susceptible.)

4. Reoxygenation of hypoxic cells. (This is particularly important because tumors develop poorly oxygenated sections, owing to blood supply problems, as their size increases beyond a few cubic micrometers, and cells exposed to radiation in the absence of oxygen are two to three times more resistant than cells exposed in the presence of oxygen.)

Nutritional approaches do not appear to have been used much to date to try to enhance radiation therapy, and little has been published even by those physicians, such as Dr. Glenn Warner in Seattle, who use them as an important component of their practice. However, there are indications from both clinical observation and animal experiments that this therapeutic ratio of effects on tumor cells versus normal cells can be beneficially manipulated, using both specific and general nutritional alterations to achieve the dual objective of (1) enhancing the tumor-destroying aspect of radiotherapy and (2) maximizing the preservation of healthy tissues with the minimum of overall distress and reaction on the part of the patient.

In addition, nutritional factors are clearly important in the long-term healing of the damaged normal tissue and in enhancing the body's natural ability to fight residual tumor cells.

Let us look more carefully at some of the more promising specific approaches and the supporting evidence.

We have discussed the roles of the antioxidants in radiation damage protection in Chapter 3. The general guidelines for utilizing these nutrients as protectors of the body against the side effects of radiation therapy must be reconsidered here with a major proviso: care must be taken that such protection does not in fact unacceptably reduce the effectiveness of the radiotherapy.

VITAMIN A

A variety of studies with vitamin A and beta-carotene are very promising; they indicate no detraction from the tumor cell–killing ability of the radiotherapy, as well as an enhancement of wound healing and survival rates.

In a study at the Albert Einstein College of Medicine, Levenson et al. (1984) showed that supplemental vitamin A prevents acute radiation-induced defects in wound healing. They showed that wounds created in laboratory rats which were subsequently irradiated (with 750 to 850 rads) healed much better if the rats had been supplemented with vitamin A, and the rats generally withstood the radiation better. The level used was 25 times the normal amount considered necessary for health in rats (150,000 international units of vitamin A per kilogram of body weight). Interestingly, the benefits noted in the supplemented irradiated rats, which included less weight loss, less gastric ulceration, and less unnatural blood changes, were achieved whether the rats were supplemented 2 or 4 days before the irradiation or 2 days after, with some effects up to 4 days after radiation. It is suggested that the wound-healing results were due to vitamin A's ability to increase early inflammatory reactions to wounding, stimulating healing and lessening radiation damage.

In 1959, Dr. Wolfgang Scheef, Director of the Janker Clinic in Bonn, Germany, reported that 50 patients with bronchogenic carcinoma treated with emulsified vitamin A and radiotherapy showed a 1-year survival rate of 36%, compared with a survival rate of only 9% among control subjects receiving radiotherapy alone.

VITAMIN E

Recent studies with vitamin E succinate supplementation suggest that it may be very promising in terms of significantly improving radiation therapy's therapeutic ratio (see Figure 7).

Sarria and Prasad (1984) have produced evidence in tissue culture of achieving this dual objective via supplementation with *dl*-alpha-tocopherol. They showed that vitamin E succinate markedly enhanced the effect of cobalt 60 radiation, making tumor cells more vulnerable and simultaneously acting to protect normal cells. They state that the exact mechanisms whereby vitamin E modifies radiation response is unknown but that its antioxidant properties were probably the major factor. They note that in other studies, vitamin C has been shown to increase radiation response of neuroblastoma cells in culture (cf. Prasad et al., 1979). Sarria and Prasad state, "The commonly accepted view that an antioxidant should protect tissue from radiation damage may be applicable to certain normal tissues. The fact that the administration of vitamin E before irradiation protects normal tissues supports this view. The reasons for the differential effect of vitamin E in modifying the radiation response of tumor cells and normal cells are unknown, however . . . the presence of an excess amount of antioxidant inside cells may be lethal." They go on to suggest that membrane changes may differentially affect vitamin E uptake into normal and tumor cells and allow the entry of an excess amount of vitamin E into tumor cells. Ionizing radiation would further impair this control, so that further increased amounts of vitamin E enter the cells. This, they say, may be lethal and could account for the enhancement of tissue detruction in tumor cells by radiation in the presence of vitamin E.

It becomes clear from this discussion that there is hope in meeting the dual objective in radiotherapy of finding means which not only make tumor cells more vulnerable, but are protective of normal cells or at the least do not also make them more vulnerable to radiation damage. However, the subject is complex, and a great deal of additional data collection and controlled research is still needed before the point is reached where the application to human beings is clear-cut. The trend, though, is clear and opens an exciting area of research as well as giving substantial direction and encouragement to those wishing to apply nutritional concepts in dealing with their own radiation therapy.

VITAMIN C

There are some indications that radiotherapy substantially increases the body's need for vitamin C by 300%. One must also consider that biochemical individuality creates substantial variations in individual requirements for many nutrients, including ascorbate (cf. Williams, 1979). However, a substantial question has been raised about the advisability of high-dosage supplementation with vitamin C during actual receipt of radiotherapy. This is because radiation generates free radicals in the vitamin C itself, which can these cause more harm than good. Thus, vitamin C probably should not be taken supplementally during actual radiation therapy, although it is probably advisable as soon as the therapy is completed.

GLUTATHIONE

Meister (1983) cites a number of animal studies which indicate that induced *depletion* of glutathone prior to radiation therapy leads to tissues being more amenable to destruction. It has long been known, he states, that irradiation leads to decrease in cellular glutathione which, when present, protects against the effects of radiation. He suggests that the manipulation of glutathione metabolism, by use of enzyme inhibitors, for example, should be done in order to decrease its active presence in the body during radiotherapy (or chemotherapy), thus reducing its defensive capability and enhancing the therapeutic destruction of tumor cells. (Again, this emphasizes the complexity of the problems in dealing with radiation therapy.) He emphasizes that this need not have deleterious effects on other nontreated cells, since their SOD activity would still help provide protection. Meister's work thus suggests that supplementation with anything which would enhance glutathione activity might be undesirable during radiation therapy; such substances are discussed in Chapter 3. They should be resumed after such treatment to boost antioxidant and antitumor activity.

AN ENCOURAGING FIELD TRIAL

Professor Emeritus Emanuel Cheraskin of the University of Alabama investigated the possibility of both improving the degree of response to radiotherapy and minimizing negative effects (Cheraskin et al., 1968). He explains, "The impact of ionizing radiation may be conveniently considered in two categories: (1) the direct effect on tumor cells, and (2) the indirect effect on the tumor, mediated through alterations in the host and the tumor bed." The success of radiotherapy is measured by the product of both of these body changes. When the clinician decides whether or not radiotherapy has been successful, both characteristics of the tumor itself, as well as characteristics of the person who has the tumor, are considered, in order to monitor results and for prediction of the likely outcome of therapy.

Cheraskin and his co-workers examined the radiation response in matched groups of patients with cervical cancer. One group received specialized dietary advice (relatively high protein, low refined carbohydrate, together with multimineral and multivitamin supplementation), while a control group irradiated at the same time received no dietary advice. The dietary program commenced 1 week prior to radiotherapy and continued until 3 weeks after cessation of therapy. It consisted of the following:

Animal protein such as fish, meat, fowl, and eggs was encouraged at each meal.

Carbohydrates of low nutritional value, such as snacks, desserts, white flour, and all sugar were eliminated. Complex carbohydrates were encouraged.

Multivitamin-multimineral supplements (one Abbott Optilets-M) were used, which provided 500 milligrams vitamin C, 100 milligrams niacinamide, 20 milligrams calcium pantothenate, 15 milligrams vitamin B_1, 10 milligrams B_2, 5 milligrams B_6, 10,000 IU vitamin A, 12 micrograms vitamin B_{12}, 400 IU vitamin D, 30 IU vitamin E, 80 milligrams magnesium, 20 milligrams iron, 2 milligrams copper, 1.5 milligrams zinc, 1 milligram manganese, 0.15 milligrams iodine; plus two Duo-CVP ascorbic acid–bioflavonoid capsules. The reasoning was that this would allow optimal intake of nutrient-rich foods. The multivitamin-multimineral supplements were given to provide nutrients in excess of normally accepted levels of requirement, particularly for antioxidants.

The results were very encouraging. Those receiving no advice on diet (30 subjects) had an average positive response of 63.3%. This is regarded as poor; the standard point at which a response is thought of as "good," 70%, was achieved by only half of the women. Of the nearly 30 women receiving radiotherapy who followed the dietary advice, the average response was 93.5%. This group had no poor responders, and the average was derived from a lowest response of 91% to a highest of 100%. This latter "perfect score" was achieved by many of these patients. Every patient in the dietary group demonstrated a favorable score using standard medical criteria for analyzing the response rate to radiotherapy. The researchers commented that among those who received no nutritional advice, while the average was poor and indeed over half had very poor results, there were some good responders. They suggest that this may have been related to their own normal nutritional habits, but unfortunately no data were collected.

Cheraskin's study indicates a marked contrast between the groups. It appears that similar studies could be mounted to confirm the efficacy of optimum nutrition with relatively little expense or effort and would certainly not subject the patients to any increased risk; it is difficult to understand why there have not been more follow-up studies in the intervening period. Even partial confirmation of this study would be expected to result in practices that increase the benefits of radiotherapy greatly and enhance the comfort and well-being of patients undergoing this stressful experience.

EFFECTS OF RADIOTHERAPY ON NUTRITIONAL STATUS

A number of factors determine the degree of nutritionally related problems experienced by the patient undergoing radiation therapy. These include (1) the part of the body irradiated, (2) the intensity of the radiation, (3) the time over which radiation is administered, (4) the volume of tissue treated, and (5) the prior nutritional status of the patient. As has already been mentioned, most patients receiving high-dose irradiation of the head, neck, abdomen, or pelvis lose at least 10% of their body weight during a 6–8 week course of treatment, and the problem is compounded by the fact that most of the patients are malnourished before treatment starts.

Many aspects of the problem need to be considered.

If the head and neck are irradiated, side effects often include dry mouth, swallowing difficulties, and eventual dental decay as a result of underproduction of saliva and mucus; loss of taste and smell; sore mouth with burning sensations; and ulcerations that make swallowing painful. The patient receiving irradiation of the esophagus also experiences swallowing difficulties due to mucosal damage, formation of fibrous tissue narrowing the passageway, and/or nerve damage. Irradiation of the abdomen and pelvis can lead to nausea, vomiting, and diarrhea. Absorption of nutrients is impaired by damage to the intestinal mucosa: flattening of villi, decrease in digestive enzymes, narrowing of the passage, and ulceration and inflammation of small blood vessels. Some of these problems may continue over months or years. The resultant diarrhea can further lead to loss of water and electrolytes.

All of this implies that it is essential that the patient be in as good a nutritional state as possible prior to radiation therapy, that the patient be given excellent nutritional support during therapy in ways that can be used by the particular individual (in addition to using the specific radioprotective approaches, already discussed), and that the person be carefully monitored and supported nutritionally for an extended time after the end of radiation treatment. These factors are reviewed very well by Booker (1983). Dr. Edward Copeland, then Professor of Surgery at the University of Texas Medical School, has shown that a hyperalimentation diet (optimum feeding) was successful in replenishing the strength of cancer patients receiving both chemotherapy and radiotherapy (Copeland, 1977 and 1979).

One area in which nutritional supplementation has clear desirability is that of prevention of nausea, which is frequent following radiotherapy. It is standard medical practice to provide vitamin B_6 to anyone with such symptoms, and many radiologists now provide it before treatment as a preventive measure, which seems a sensible approach. In the dosages required, 50 to 150 milligrams, pyridoxine is perfectly safe.

Protection of tissues from damage during receipt of radiotherapy and overall enhancement of quality of life has been attempted by a variety of methods. German studies by Hernuss et al. (1975) involved female patients receiving cobalt 60 irradiation for the treatment of inoperable cancers. Some were given 20 grams daily of pollen, whereas a control group received no supplementation prior to radiotherapy. A variety of beneficial effects were noted among those receiving the pollen, including a 50% reduction in nausea, improved appetite, fewer sleep disturbances, reduced inflammation, and a variety of indications in blood status of a greater degree of normality than was the case in the control group. The overall rate of decline in their health was reduced to a third of the rate in the controls. No conclusions were reached as to what constituent(s) in pollen offered these benefits, but the report indicates the possibility of enhancement of overall quality of life in advanced cancer patients receiving radiotherapy.

At this point, it is too early to detail a complete regimen for those undergoing radiation therapy, and there will clearly be differences depending on the details of the cancer, the treatment protocol, and the general health of the patient. However, there is much hope, and many clear suggestions at this point can be made, chiefly the diet used by Cheraskin, with particular attention to vitamin A, beta-carotenes, vitamin E, vitamin B_6, general nutritional support, and perhaps bee pollen.

CHAPTER SIX

EXCLUDING THE TROJAN HORSE:
Nutritional Removal of Radioactive Material From the Body

Up to this point, we have discussed ways of dealing with ionizing radiation impinging upon the body from the outside. Here, we talk about a special situation in which we are forced to deal with a potential enemy *within* – atoms that can enter and become incorporated into the very structures of our bodies, like a Trojan horse. They then decay there over weeks, months, or years, giving off ionizing radiation and potentially causing damage. These are radioisotopes, close relatives of normal elements in our bodies, which are, however, unstable or radioactive, as discussed in Chapter 1. They include iodine 131, strontium 90, cesium 137, potassium 40, and carbon 14. They are always present in very low levels in our environment but only become of significance when the intense energies of a nuclear explosion or reactor lead to their production in large amounts and their release into the environment. Chernobyl is a major case in point; in this most catastrophic nuclear accident to date, high levels of these isotopes were dumped over most of western Europe, giving levels of radioactivity in people's lawns substantially above those that would normally be found in many scientists' laboratories. In many areas, some of these radioisotopes will remain in the soil for years to come, continuing to enter the food chain and to potentially cause contamination in other ways.

It makes sense for us to attempt to block the entry of these radioactive materials into our bodies and to eliminate as much radioactive material as possible that may have already entered, before it can do additional harm. This attempt should be in addition to the sorts of measures discussed in Chapters 3 and 4 to deal with the direct effects of the radiation as it is produced by residual radioactive material.

Clearly, the best initial approach is to develop sensible patterns of behavior to avoid contact with radioactive materials which might be present in the environment, atmosphere, or food. Our first line of defense is political: the probability of nuclear contamination is decreased by reducing nuclear armaments, insisting on strong reactor safety measures and excellent training of personnel, pushing research on soil decontamination techniques, and being sure that there would be strong public warning in the case of any significant radiation leak. During any period of heavy contamination, such as happened after Chernobyl, prudence would include avoiding going out in the rain (which brings down radioactive materials in the air), using care in handling outdoor garments, not letting small children play in grass or sandboxes, washing hands and vegetables carefully, avoiding leafy vegetables, and not letting farm animals—particularly milk producers—graze outdoors. Such measures were adopted widely in much of Germany and Scandinavia after Chernobyl, while no such warnings were generally issued in France, reflecting political expediencies and differing interpretations of "safe" levels. In effect, a massive experiment was thus conducted on the effectiveness of such measures, if we havé the wisdom to carefully collect and analyze the data over the next 30 years.

The next line of defense is the digestive system, the major region through which radioisotopes entering the body are likely to travel. This should receive attention in an attempt to dislodge unwelcome radioactive material brought in through contaminated food or drink. The approach should also help eliminate much that might have already been absorbed into the system and be passing from the liver into the digestive tract carried in the bile. The bile and most of its constituents—including any radio-active salts—are then reabsorbed, along with the dietary fats, which the soap-like bile has broken up into small globules that are usable. Nutritional tricks can help prevent this reuptake of unwanted minerals, including radioisotopes, and also of choles-terol, a bonus for people for whom that is a problem. Strontium 90, iodine 131, and cesium 137 are the forms of radioactive material most likely to enter the body as a result of nuclear accidents. Iodine 131 has a short half-life—only 8 days—so in its case, the direct problems (and appropriate counter-measures) are short-lived. However, strontium 90 and cesium 137 are likely to find their way into the topsoil of an area thus affected, and it takes decades for them to decay. Thus, once an area has been contaminated, careful monitoring of soil and produce is important, and the prevention programs outlined in this book may be desirable for years in order to minimize the longterm risks. One further complication is that levels may vary as much as 30-fold within a few miles of each other after major global releases, as is seen in southern Germany after Chernobyl, de-pending on vagaries of wind and timing of rainfall. Similar factors can also lead to sporadic episodes of very high localized fallout, such as that from a Nevada nuclear test which was brought down by rain over Albany and Troy, New York, in April 1953. This general topic is very well discussed by Sternglass (1986), along with the health implications of low-level radioactivity.

Radioactive material absorbed into the body via food or through inhalation circulates throughout the body via the blood-stream. Some is likely to become bound to favored sites, such as the bones for cesium and strontium, which are chemically similar to calcium; and the thyroid gland for iodine 137, which becomes incorporated, like other iodine, into thyroid hormones.

It is while these radioactive materials are still in the digestive tract that we have the best opportunity to introduce substances which can bind them selectively or compete for their uptake out of the intestine and can thus assist in their safe elimination from the body. We will next discuss some of the most effective of these.

PECTIN

Pectin is a kind of fiber found in many fruits and vegetables and is particularly abundant in apples and sunflower seeds. It is familiar to those of you who make jams and jellies as the ingredient used to thicken and solidify them. It is quite unlike the fiber in grain bran or most other fibers, in that it is soluble in hot water and forms a gel when cooling. It binds cations, including the radioisotopes discussed above, and also speeds transit time through the gut. The potentially problematic materials are then excreted in the stool. A number of experiments have indicated pectin's usefulness during radiation exposure.

Under most circumstances, sufficient pectin should be obtained by eating six apples a day and/or several ounces of sunflower seeds; this may be doubled under acute conditions. Other good sources of pectin include oranges, grapefruit, grapes, and berries. Pectin is also available in tablet form, sometimes combined with acidophilus for repopulating the digestive system with healthy bacteria. The pectin intake should be spread out over the day to keep a continued presence in the bowel to bind any passing radioisotope. A high-pectin regimen has other health benefits. It helps remove heavy metals, such as aluminum, cadmium, and lead, functioning as a natural chelating agent, and aids the elimination of bile acids from the digestive system, lowering serum cholesterol.

ALGIN AND KELP

The mucilaginous fiber algin, which is derived from seaweed, is completely indigestible. It has an affinity for such minerals as strontium and cesium as well as for heavy metals, acting like pectin to speed their transit through the digestive tract, decrease their absorption, and excrete them with bowel movements.

Russian research in this field is particularly intense. For example, Danetskaia et al. (1977) administered cesium 137 and strontium 90 to rats, either in single exposures or on a continued schedule. Calcium, sodium alginate, and Prussian blue were used in doses of 258, 800, and 50 milligrams per rat per day for the experimental group, and life expectancy and cancer development were compared with those in a parallel control group without these supplements. A protective effect was noted whenever there was chronic exposure. There were half the number of cancerous growths, with survival considerably extended (by 120 days) when algin, calcium, and Prussian blue were being used. In the protected animals there was a 17-fold reduction in cesium absorbed, and a four-fold reduction in strontium in the skeleton.

Algin is readily available in the form of sodium alginate in powder form or in half-gram doses. About 10 grams (2 tablespoons) per day, in divided doses for the duration of exposure, should produce similar results to those noted in the animal studies. This is also an almost certain cure for low-fiber–induced constipation, as the gel-like bulk of the algin will ensure normal bowel health. At this point, alginate is purified from seaweed. However, the alginate gene has recently been cloned using recombinant DNA techniques (Deretic et al., 1987), so it should soon be possible to produce this important polysaccharide in pure form and limitless quantity from high-yielding bacterial strains. The eating of seaweed such as dried Japanese komba, nori, hijiki, arame, or wakame (among others), which are available from specialist and oriental shops, also offers a fine source of algin, although it is harder to quantitate. Such kelp can be eaten as a vegetable or incorporated into soups or stews. Kelp powder and tablets are also available, although the amount of algin in them is not always stated, and very high doses may be required.

Algin is sometimes sold in combination with selenium, as selenium alginate. For example, Larkhall Laboratories makes a formula which combines 50 micrograms of selenium with 500 milligrams of algin and additional vitamin B_6, vitamin E, magnesium, and lecithin, all of which are useful in antiradiation protocols. However, there is a danger of excessive selenium if high doses of this are taken; not more than four selenium alginate tablets should be taken daily for longer than a week. Possibly, other sources of algin should be used as well if this approach is taken.

Since algin remains undigested by the body, it has no inherent toxic limit. However, absorption of essential minerals like zinc and calcium can also be reduced, so high levels should not be used indiscriminately or indefinitely, and the body's needs for the other metals must be taken into consideration.

IODINE

Another advantage of using seaweed, as a food or powder or as kelp tablets, is that it provides a good source of iodine. This competes with radioactive iodine 131 for intake into the thyroid, where the iodine 131 can cause devastating damage, as it is selectively concentrated and incorporated into the thyroid hormones.

Excessive iodine consumption can be problematic, but the level provided by the kelp suggested above is still reasonable. Supplements such as Lambert's Pacific Kelp provide 150 micrograms per tablet, so ten tablets provide about 15 times the RDA for iodine of 150 micrograms. Studies by Ringsdorf and Cheraskin (1980) strongly suggest that this is still within safe and possibly even advantageous levels. They analyzed the iodine intake of over 1000 doctors and found a range of 100 to 4,500 micrograms, with an average of 500 micrograms. Using the Cornell Medical Index questionnaire, he also surveyed these doctors for a total of over 200 health-related symptoms. He found that the number of symptoms noted was inversely correlated with the iodine intake up to at least 1000 micrograms per day; the higher the intake, the fewer the symptoms. Thus, 1500 micrograms per day should give substantial protection without significant risk during periods of some exposure to iodine 131. (Incidentally, similar results were found for a number of other nutrients for levels up to approximately 10 times their RDAs, as well, which is encouraging in thinking about using protective supplementation.) For acute exposure, as was experienced in some areas after Chernobyl, higher amounts could be needed— up to 50 milligrams for up to two weeks—but such levels can suppress thyroid function and should be used only with great caution and attention to symptoms of thyroid problems.

Chernobyl even had some unexpected benefits. After the accident there, Italians were issued iodized salt to help protect against the iodine 131 to which they were being exposed. The babies born of mothers using the iodized salt were found to have significantly fewer thyroid problems than were normally found in that population—a good argument for the iodine supplementation of salt to be continued, as is routinely done in the United States.

CALCIUM AND MAGNESIUM

As mentioned earlier, the chemical properties of calcium are quite similar to those of strontium and cesium. If calcium is present in high levels, it very effectively competes with both radioisotopes for uptake out of the bowel into the bloodstream, as well as for later deposit into the bone. The same factor makes calcium useful in dealing with contamination by such heavy metals as lead and mercury.

A variety of rich natural sources of calcium, such as green vegetables and apples, also are good sources of other helpful nutrients. Fresh milk should, however, be viewed with suspicion in times of radioactive fallout, since it is particularly vulnerable to contamination, especially if the cows are grazing outdoors. For example, by the time the children of Levlev, 5.6 miles from Chernobyl, were evacuated 2–3 days after the accident, radiation in their thyroids already measured as high as 250 rem, the result of iodine 131 which had already managed to get from the grass into their milk, and much milk throughout western Europe was also very highly contaminated (Edwards, 1987).

At least 1500 milligrams of calcium a day, divided into at least four doses, should probably be ingested during times of exposure to significant quantities of radionucleotides. This situation almost certainly requires supplementation. Bone meal, from the long bones of cattle, is an excellent source, since it combines calcium with magnesium and phosphorus in appropriate balance. Dolomite should generally be avoided, since it has been shown to frequently be contaminated with unacceptable levels of lead. Research since the 1950s has demonstrated the usefulness of this approach.

CLAY

Clay has well-known adsorptive properties. As described in the *Dispensatory of the United States*, "in aqueous suspensions, the individual particles of clay (bentonite) are negatively charged, thus resulting in a strong attraction for positively charged ions, and being responsible for its clarifying liquid containing positively charged particles of suspended matter. In addition to the growing number of external uses for bentonite, it is reported to be of value as an intestinal evacuent when in the form of a gel." As with algin and pectin, a variety of studies have demonstrated the ability of clay to help eliminate such positive radioisotopes as strontium and cesium, along with toxic heavy metals, and the material is not absorbed. However, it should not be taken regularly for longer than a month. Aluminum oxide is a major component of clay, so even very low amounts of absorption could provide problem levels of aluminum over the long term. There is again the potential problem of its also binding useful trace minerals like zinc and calcium, so similar precautions apply.

Clay comes in a variety of forms. Bentonite is widely available in the United States and is used for dealing with many kinds of poisoning. The French are devoted to fine green clay — argilla vert surfine. It may be taken as a suspension in water, starting with just the liquid left on top a few hours after a teaspoonful is put into a half glass of water. Later, more of the powder is taken as well, or the clay may be taken in very small pellets, made by moistening the powder and rolling it into pellets which are then baked in an oven. The flavor can be greatly improved by including a herblike mint in the paste. The normal time for taking clay is half an hour or so before meals, particularly breakfast; in cases of extreme exposure, it should be taken three times a day. Liquid intake should be increased substantially, especially if there is initial constipation.

VITAMIN E

There is evidence that vitamin E may play a very useful role in coping with radioactive material in the intestinal tract, in addition to its general systemic antioxidant role discussed earlier. Specifically, it may help reduce the damage to the colon tissue itself caused by radioactive material–induced free radical production in the intestine. This has been studied particularly for chemical producers of free radicals, such as dimethylhydrazine. Cook and McNamara (1980) showed that the frequency of colorectal carcinomas and adenomas was very substantially reduced by including high levels of vitamin E in the diet (600 vs. 10 milligrams per kilogram of body weight, with no other differences in the diets). Beckman et al. (1982) showed an encouraging reduction of radiation-induced lethal mutations by vitamin E, which would help explain the mechanism involved here.

ACIDOPHILUS

The methods used to remove radioactive material from the intestinal tract, and also the damage to the gut from the radiation, will tend to upset the normal ecological balance of microorganisms there. Thus, it is wise to use live yogurt, drink acidophilus milk, and probably supplement with a good-quality acidophilus powder preparation, such as Superdophilus, to restore a healthy microbial balance in the gut and thus enhance the body's general homeostasis.

CHAPTER SEVEN

THE INVISIBLE ENEMY:
Sources of Radioactivity

We are constantly exposed to radiation, both ionizing and non-ionizing, and the amount to which we are exposed is likely to increase. Nuclear power will undoubtedly take a significant part of the burden of supplying energy in the foreseeable future. Coal is plentiful in most areas, but the anxieties and real damage resulting from acid rain, which is almost certainly a by-product of the burning of fossil fuels such as coal, makes its long-term use in energy production unlikely. In addition, significant quantities of radioactive carbon 14 are released when coal is burned, and those who mine it pay a high price in terms of damage to their lungs and other aspects of their health. Oil will decline in supply over the next decades, and in most parts of the world, development of power from such renewable resources as the sun, wind, and tides has been slow and expensive. Thus, nuclear reactors are likely to be called upon to meet the power needs of industrial nations to a substantial degree for a long time to come. In this regard, it is particularly important for the public to become familiar with such issues as those discussed recently in "Hanford's Radioactive Tumbleweed" (Marshall, 1987) and by Wilson (1987).

Safer reactors will undoubtedly be developed, and some are already in existence in prototype forms. These will reduce the dangers of current water-cooled reactors, by replacing water with gas, by altering the way in which water is used as a coolant, or by quite different technologies. It is hoped that radiation contamination of the environment from such reactors will become even less a danger than is the case with current methods of nuclear power generation. However, nuclear weapons testing will continue in all probability, adding to overall background radiation levels.

Most everyday hazards of radiation are not, however, related to such large-scale happenings as weapon testing or reactor explosions and leaks. They are far closer to home, as was briefly outlined in Chapter 1.

Some of the avoidable and unavoidable dangers will be summarized here. Let us start by recalling that the danger to health and life relating to a given contact with radioactive material depends not only on the properties of the substance but on its chemistry. For example, radioactive iodine 131, washing onto you during a walk in the rain, presents little health danger, whereas eating food contaminated with this same radioactive substance will ensure that it reaches your thyroid and thus is capable of doing great harm.

The amount of harm which accrues also depends upon the size of the dose. There is no safe level, however, as discussed in Chapter 1. When a substance is radioactive, its atomic nuclei are disintegrating, and it is this which causes the emission of particles (or waves) of ionizing energy. There are a surprising number of sources of such energy.

David Poch, in his book *Radiation Alert,* catalogues the major sources of radiation danger in everyday life, and quite a catalogue it is:

Building materials: Approximately one third of the natural radiation to which we are exposed comes from radon gas, which is a decay product of uranium. It is found naturally in many rock formations and gradually released over long periods of time; it is noted in houses built of granite or sometimes brick or concrete. Homes thus constructed have 50% more radon contamination than do those built of wood. The potentially serious effects of radon in homes and buildings was recently discussed by Doege and Hendee (1987); unlike other forms of radiation, radon contamination seems to do more harm in constant small doses than in large one-time exposures.

Phospho-gypsum, a building material derived from by-products of the mining for fertilizer of phosphate rock, is highly radioactive and should be avoided. A comparative study of building material shows that granite contains an average of 4.7 parts per million (ppm) uranium and 2.0 ppm thorium. Cement contains about 3.4 ppm uranium and 5.1 ppm thorium. Manufactured anhydride, a by-product of gypsum, contains 13.7 ppm uranium and 16.1 ppm thorium. By comparison, sandstone contains only about 0.45 ppm uranium and 1.7 ppm thorium.

Occasionally, problems are caused by radon gas leaking from the bedrock under homes; such difficulties have been reported in the news repeatedly in recent years. (Suspected leaks can be investigated by local or state officials.) Water deriving from sources which bring it into contact with radioactive rock often carries radon gas, which becomes airborne eventually, when taps are run or showers used. It is then easily inhaled. Water passing through rock and derived from wells is higher in radon than that from lakes or reservoirs.

Contamination by radon, like that by some other pollutants, has become a greater problem with the recent emphasis on tight insulation of homes with very little airflow out; the problem can be reduced by regular, thorough airing out.

Ceramics: Many items of tableware and decorative glassware contain uranium compounds. Some contain as high as 20% uranium oxide. This produces high-energy gamma and beta radiation and can be deposited in the internal organs of the body when acidic foods placed in such ceramics leach out these compounds. The dose of radiation possible from this source is high if it is used frequently, possibly exceeding the annual radiation limits thought to be acceptable from all sources. Those glazes most likely to be contaminated in this way are characterized by a bright, shiny, reflective surface, often in orangey-red, beige, or yellow. State or local health authorities could be asked to test doubtful ceramic tableware.

Cigarettes: We have already mentioned this source of radioactivity. The tobacco leaf is commonly found to be a source of radioactive lead 210 or polonium 210, which, it is thought, may derive from phosphate-based fertilizers used in tobacco growing. Alpha radiation derives from the radioactive lead and from the polonium, which is itself a decay product of the lead (as is another, less hazardous substance, radioactive bismuth 210). These decay products are thought to dissolve in the lungs and to be cleared away, but this is not true of the radioactive lead itself. It can remain in the lungs for years, or it can migrate to other tissues, particularly bone, emitting radiation all the time. As you may remember, alpha radiation is effective only over a fairly short distance, but it causes intense damage in that region because of the large size of the very energetic alpha particles involved.

Optical glass: This is often a source of radioactivity, since the rare earths used in its manufacture often contain radioactive thorium or uranium. Radiation from spectacles would be small but constant, and is thought to relate to cataract development. Plastic lenses are not radioactive.

Camper's lamps: The white mantle found in camping lamps contains thorium, a radioactive substance which gives off highly charged alpha particles. Thorium eventually decays to form radium 228, which in turn becomes radon 220, all of which produce alpha radiation. Emission is highest soon after the lighting of the lamp, and so this should be done outdoors and the lamp left for 20 minutes or so before being brought into a confined space. Care is also suggested in changing mantles. In particular, hands should be washed carefully afterwards before handling food, and the lamp should if possible be in a well-ventilated place, since alpha particles are a problem only if they are ingested or breathed into the lungs.

Fertilizers: Many sources of fertilizer are radioactive. These include phosphate rock, the source of phosphorus which is used widely in farming and horticulture. This contains uranium and its breakdown products, which find their ways into the end product. (As mentioned earlier, tobacco is thought to become radioactive via this source.)

Smoke detectors: These are commonly found in public buildings, stores, hotels, and many private homes. Some forms have an ionization chamber in their construction, which avoids the potential problem of a battery running out. When this is so, the appliance should carry a warning about radioactive material inside it. If airtight, it is safe; if not, gamma radiation will be emitted. The greatest danger would occur during a fire, where exposure to the core material, americium 241, could occur. Many other fire detectors use different technology and are not potential radiation risks.

Color television sets and video display units: Color TVs and VDUs may emit x-rays. This is far more likely in older color TV sets, in which x-ray emission was readily measurable. Modern solid-state sets have a lower potential for this. Nevertheless, sitting close to a color VDU or TV set is unwise. Remember that children are more sensitive to radiation damage than are adults. Public video game parlors represent a risk to young people inasmuch as some TV screens leak radiation and thus expose the players and viewers to its effects.

Watch dials: Radium is used on the luminous dials of watches and clocks, and these should be avoided. (Some of the earliest evidence that radiation is carcinogenic came from the very high incidence of mouth cancers in watch-dial painters, who traditionally licked their brushes to bring them to a very fine point.)

ULTRAVIOLET RADIATION

Ultraviolet radiation can cause sunburn, eye damage, skin cancer, and other long-term damage. The potential dangers from this source are discussed in some detail in Chapters 1 and 2, and lead to the unavoidable conclusion that unnecessary exposure to sunlight and other UV sources should be avoided.

NONIONIZING RADIATION

This is not the major concern of this book, which is aimed at providing information about protection against ionizing, high-energy radioactivity, but it still should be mentioned here. Low-energy nonionizing radiation surrounds us from cradle to grave, and its effects are quite different from the dangers described, although in some cases the potential for harm is also great. As David Poch puts it in *Radiation Alert,* "At the dose level we typically experience in the environment (for example from telecommunications) or in the home (from microwave ovens) or in the workplace (from video display units) low energy forms of radiation do not result in immediately identifiable damage to the cells of our bodies. The primary concern with doses of low-energy radiation is the possibility of subtle effects on our nervous system and the chemical 'communications systems' within our bodies, that regulate virtually every bodily function."

He notes that while there may be a connection between low-energy radiation and cancer or genetic effects, we do not know enough about this as yet to estimate the risks. The form of the

radiation appears to be important, i.e., whether pulsed or continuous, pulsed forms being more damaging. We know little about
the effects of high-voltage electricity transmission on people living under, or near, transmission lines, apart from repeated
reports of increased degrees of ill health. Biological effects on
animals and plants have been noted, but little is certain about
how these effects are taking place.

It is known from the work of John Ott (1982) that such
apparently safe radiation sources as fluorescent light damage the
health. Since these emit (in the main) light which does not
correspond with the full spectrum found in natural sunlight, the
effect is different from that of daylight. This is noted in plants
(which will not easily bloom in artificial light unless a full spectrum is provided) and chickens in broiler houses (where the
addition of full-spectrum strip lighting dramatically alters their
disease rate and laying capacity). He also reports experiments
suggesting that hyperactive children who displayed aggressive
tendencies in school were turned into calmer beings by the
altering of strip lighting in their classes, from conventional to full-
spectrum.

We know little of the long-term consequences of our interaction with the multitude of radiation sources, both low- and high-
energy, which surround us in our modern world. The various
kinds of radiation are described in Chapter 1. What are the
effects of radiowaves, microwaves, infrared light, or even visible
light — the only radiation we can see? What are the long-term
hazards of irradiated foods? What we do know may be summarized thus:

Extremely low-frequency radiation (from electric power lines,
VDUs, etc.) is nonionizing radiation. This is a possible carcinogen, but the overall health-damaging effects are not understood
as yet. It appears that people's behavior is affected by such
radiation.

Radio waves. Also nonionizing, these appear to disrupt physiological processes including the cardiovascular system.

Microwaves, which are also nonionizing, can at low levels
disrupt physiological processes and at high levels raise body
temperature and cause cataracts. They may be released from
old-model or, in some cases, defective microwave ovens and
have also been used for certain communication purposes.

Infrared radiation at high levels raises body temperature.

Visible light can cause eye damage and raise body temperature under some circumstances. However, too little light can cause as great a problem. This is particularly true for people suffering from S.A.D. (seasonal affective disorder.) Such people experience a profound depression in the winter, which we know is reversible simply by exposure to a battery of full-spectrum lights for several hours a day.

There is significant evidence that *irradiated food,* while not itself radioactive, has suffered nutritional damage, especially in vitamin E, and contains many unidentified radiological products ("urps"), the biological effects of which are unknown. For an excellent, detailed recent treatment of the subject, we refer you to Webb, Lang, and Tucker, *Food Irradiation: Who Wants It?*

We also have evidence of the effects of earth radiation in more subtle ways, where the so called ley-lines of the earth's electromagnetic discharge appear to influence the health of people living above them. Underground streams alter the electromagnetic energy in the overlying land, and health patterns seem to be different in consequence, showing a higher incidence of cancer, for example, in people living there.

Much remains to be understood regarding the subtle influences of radiation and electromagnetism on the human body. By no means are all such influences harmful. Bones have been made to knit more rapidly when electromagnetic energy is applied to them. Scans of the body using magnetic resonance will prove safer than x-radiation. What we have ascertained is that it will pay dividends to monitor the environment, to alter it accordingly where this seems beneficial, and, where possible, to keep careful epidemiological records of health patterns and to take protective measures which are available through nutritional and other means.

MONITORING THE ENVIRONMENT

One method is to use a radiation detection device, as discussed in Chapter 1. A personal Geiger counter might be a reasonable safeguard, through which local levels of gamma and the more energetic beta radiation may be checked, although they are not very sensitive. There are many different versions which will give information on various ranges of radioactivity. Some have alarms which are preset to warn against high levels. These can be used to monitor food, pets, water, buildings, soil, etc. in emergency situations but are of little use with the normal low-level radiation to which we are exposed. They range in price from under $100 to much more, and, as in all things, you get what you pay for in terms of reliability and accuracy. Personal dosimeters are also available. These are commonly used by people working in exposed situations (medical staff in radiotherapy units, for example). The meters are worn on the body like a fountain pen and indicate how much radiation the person has been exposed to. They require regular analysis and recharging in order to reset them periodically. These are not inexpensive but are advisable for those in contact with radioactive materials.

A similar dosimeter is available for ultraviolet exposure to indicate damaging levels of sunlight. These can be modified to take account of skin type, indicating when a maximum degree of solar radiation has been reached.

Microwave radiation detection monitors for microwave ovens are available and inexpensive.

Thus, different types of radiation monitors can offer a degree of early warning of overexposure potential. It would be unwise, however, to allow anxiety over radiation to so dominate life as to make it an obsessive factor.

For people living near a nuclear power plant, periodic monitoring of water, soil, and food is a sensible precaution. Emphasizing the need for vigilance are the recent Freedom-of-Information Act disclosures regarding the release of a wide range of radioactive materials from and soil contamination around the Hanford Nuclear Reservation in Southeastern Washington (see Marshall, 1987). Soil which has been contaminated by radioactivity presents a problem. Russian efforts to normalize the soil in the Chernobyl area have highlighted the methods currently available. Some of these are discussed in an understandable fashion by Edwards in the April 1987 *National Geographic*. Experts in this endeavor, from the Institute of Botany at the Ukranian Academy of Sciences, also suggested that they plant lupines in the soil, as this plant absorbs radioactive elements from the earth. The ultimate disposal of the lupines, however, was thought to present another contamination problem, which ruled this method out. More suitable was the idea of irrigating the land with water to which had been added soluble calcium. This calcium would bind to much of the radioactive material and carry it down to a safe level, below crop roots. This method can be seen to have much in common with the method suggested for humans in Chapter 6, by which calcium is used to bind to radioactive materials in the bowel.

A further suggestion of the scientists would be for a combination of ash and lime to be used as fertilizer before turning the topsoil. The radioactive elements would, it is suggested, then be more likely to stay below the topsoil and not rise to the surface again.

Background radiation is constantly with us and has been throughout our evolution. We must not allow attention to its every aspect to keep us from getting on with the primary objectives of living life to the full. The overall message of this book is that the more we understand radiation the better protected we can be; there are helpful measures that can be taken either to meet specific known dangers in radiation or to have general protective effects against the many hidden sources of radiation which affect each of us. There is no suggestion that total protection is available by behavioral or nutritional measures alone. However, the many trials on animals, and the human experiences, indicate clearly that a significant degree of protection is possible. Furthermore, most of the appropriate routine nutritional protective measures are highly consistent with dietary patterns that have been shown in a variety of ways to lead to better overall health and lower incidences of such lifestyle diseases as cancer and cardiovascular problems. Their protective potential against radiation effects is just one more reason to consider their implementation. These measures are discussed in some detail in Chapters 3 and 6 and summarized in the Appendix.

APPENDIX

SUMMARY OF RADIATION PROTECTION METHODS

There now is strong supporting evidence from researchers in many lands which shows us that significant protection from the harmful effects of ionizing radiation is possible. This involves developing some understanding of the extent and nature of the hazards from various kinds of radiation, and making careful, informed choices in many aspects of behavior, as discussed in this book. In the case of unavoidable exposure to significant amounts of radiation, nutritional methods can be of assistance. These involve combining a good dietary pattern with special supplemental nutrients capable of inactivating free radicals and highly reactive oxidation products, and enhancing tissue repair. In the case of exposure to radioactive materials, it involves the reducing of the probability of their entering into the body and accelerating the removal of those that have already gained entrance.

We summarize here the mechanisms involved and the levels suggested as useful by research to date for a variety of potentially helpful agents. In many cases, much more research is still needed, and we strongly encourage you to read the appropriate sections of the book and to continue to keep informed of new research findings. Clearly, it is unreasonable to try to consume all of these potentially helpful agents, and you will generally simply choose those most appropriate to your situation.

In general, a high-protein diet that avoids fats and simple carbohydrates and provides ample trace nutrients has the potential to enhance protection from radiation damage and possibly even enhance radiation therapy effects (cf. Cheraskin study, see page 64). Particularly desirable foods include garlic, onions, cabbage, broccoli, cauliflower, citrus and other fresh foods, seeds of all sorts, cold-pressed oils, cold-water ocean fish, eggs, soured milk products, seaweeds, mushrooms, and lean meats or organ meats (avoiding fats).

The most important radiation-protective agents, acting mainly via their action as antioxidants, are the following:

Beta-carotene, 25–40 milligrams daily. (This is preferable to vitamin A, of which it is the precursor, because of its lack of toxicity and enhanced antioxidant activity.)

Vitamin E, 400–800 international units daily in water-miscible form.

Vitamin C, 500–3000 milligrams daily, in divided doses, possibly increasing to bowel tolerance in periods of strong exposure.

Selenium, 400 micrograms daily.

Nutrients important primarily due to their ability to enhance tissue integrity, the immune system, and wound healing include:

Bioflavonoids, 1–2 grams daily, with the vitamin C.

Zinc, 15–30 milligrams daily (with copper at 1–3 grams per day).

Ginseng and/or *eleutherococcus,* 0.5–2 grams daily.

Pantothenic acid, 25–100 milligrams daily in divided doses.

Vitamin B_6, 50 milligrams 2 times daily.

Essential fatty acids (see text for discussion of different types): cold-pressed oils; fish oil extracts like maxEPA; evening primrose oil.

According to available information, these doses are safe as part of a long-term program where exposure is ongoing. They should possibly be taken along with a multivitamin-multimineral at about RDA levels to avoid imbalances from supplementing specific nutrients.

Gluthathione and/or the amino acid cysteine, at 1–3 grams a day, shows evidence of also enhancing antioxidant activity. Vitamins B_1, B_2, and B_3 are involved in antiradiation activity, though with little or no direct antioxidant role; some supplementation may well be appropriate, or brewer's yeast may be used for those with no yeast allergies, at levels of 1–3 tablespoons per day. (RNA, up to 6 grams daily, may also be included for its ability to build up uric acid in the system, which also acts as an antioxidant; see text. It should not be used by anyone predisposed to gout.)

In the case of exposure to actual radioactive materials in food or environment, as in the nuclear contamination from Chernobyl, foods with high fiber content to aid elimination from the bowel (apples, sunflower seeds, kelp are much better than cereal fiber here); can supplement with algin and/or pectin 5–10 grams daily in divided doses.

Vitamins E and *C,* and *beta-carotene* or *vitamin A* for gut protection.

Competing minerals:

Calcium, 1.5 grams daily.

Magnesium, 0.75 grams daily.(1–3 grams per day defatted bone meal is a good source of both calcium and magnesium.)

Clay or *bentonite,* 1–2 teaspoonfuls daily.

Iodine, 1.5 milligrams per day; up to 50 milligrams per day for up to one week for very high acute exposure.

or *Kelp,* 0.5–1 tablespoon daily (for algin and iodine).

Green leafy vegetables (if available uncontaminated by fallout) and cruciferous vegetables like broccoli, cauliflower, and cabbage boost fiber content, supply high levels of calcium to compete with strontium 90 for absorption from the gut, and give a very high level of available beta-carotene. Apples, all sorts of seed, and berries are particularly good sources of fiber. Fatty foods and refined carbohydrates should be avoided.

In preparation for radiation therapy of tumors, look carefully at Chapter 5; it appears that a good deal can often be done to enhance both the tumor destruction and the protection of normal tissue. During actual treatment, enhanced effectiveness is reported with supplementation: vitamin E, vitamin A, and beta-carotene. An aid in nausea is Vitamin B$_6$, 100 milligrams per day. Protects normal tissues with no adverse effects: zinc, bioflavonoids. Avoid supplementation, due to effects on therapy or radiation interactions, until just after therapy is administered: vitamin C, glutathione, cysteine, selenium. Also useful is pollen 1–5 grams daily.

It is most important that other resources of free-radical activity be minimized during radiation exposure to avoid compounding the damage and to free resources for fighting the radiation effects. Thus, particular care should be taken as far as possible to avoid smoking, pollutants, and fumes as well as foods containing additives, preservatives, and coloring during periods of radiation exposure.

GLOSSARY

Accessory Nutrients: Vital to cellular function and necessary for activating specific enzymes. Accessory nutrients are distinct from essential nutrients in that they can be produced within the body at levels which would be considered adequate for most individuals. Some deficiency diseases are associated with a dietary lack of particular accessory nutrients. Accessory nutrients may be introduced into the system through dietary supplementation or dietary sources, and may be very useful in improving health.

Adaptogen: A substance that enhances the body's own recuperative powers, homeostasis, and balancing and normalizing functions without harmful side effects, whatever the nature of the health problem. Adaptogens such as ginseng, eleutherococcus, royal jelly, and pollen have strong potential for helping to maintain and regain general health in times of severe stress, including that imposed by exposure to ionizing radiation.

Alpha Particles: Positively charged form of ionizing radiation, made up of two protons and two neutrons. They cause extensive damage over a short distance, so they are particularly harmful once incorporated into the body, but they have relatively little ability to penetrate through the skin. They can cause mutations, birth defects, and cancer.

Amino Acids: The basic building blocks, or monomers, of which all proteins are composed; most proteins contain hundreds of amino acid monomers. The amino acid sequence for each protein is highly specific, determining its structural and enzymatic properties, and is the main kind of information encoded in the DNA of our genes. Twenty different specific amino acids are used in building proteins, and several others are used for other purposes in our bodies.

Becquerel (bq): One becquerel is the amount of a radioactive element needed to produce one radioactive disintegration per second.

Beta Particles: Negatively charged form of ionizing radiation, consisting of high-speed electrons. They are of medium to high energy and can penetrate 1–2 centimeters into flesh. They can cause mutations, birth defects, and cancer.

Carcinogen: Anything which is able to initiate the production of a cancerous tumor.

Curie (Ci): One curie is the amount of radioactivity present in one gram of pure radium 286. It undergoes 37 billion disintegrations per second; i.e., one curie corresponds to 37 billion becquerels, one millicurie (mCi = 0.001 curie) equals 37 million bq, and one microcurie (μc = 0.001 mCi) is 37,000 bq.

Deoxyribonucleic Acid (DNA): An extremely long linear polymer that constitutes the genetic material of each cell and is found in the nucleus, as discussed in Ch. 2.

Essential Fatty Acids (EFAs): Membrane components which cannot be produced within the body, and are thus considered essential nutrients. These include linoleic acid, alpha-linolenic acid, eicosapentaneoic acid (EPA), and their derivatives. Essential fatty acids are the most highly unsaturated membrane components, i.e., those containing the most double bonds in their outer molecular structures. They transform into important messenger molecules carrying signals between nearby cells, and are therefore particularly important in the functioning of the immune system.

Electron: Tiny negatively charged particles, 1/1835 the size of the proton, which are in orbitals outside the nucleus of each atom and balance the electric charge. As discussed in chapter 1, these electrons are arranged in specific stable shells. To complete these shells, some kinds of atoms lose 1–3 electrons, forming a positive ion, while others gain one or more electrons, forming a negative ion.

Exponential Notation: A shorthand way of writing very large and very small numbers by writing 10 followed by an exponent that indicates the number of zeros before or after the 1. Thus, 10^3 is equal to 1000, 10^5 is 100000, 10^{-3} is 0.001 and 10^{-5} is 0.00001.

Free Radical: An atom or molecule that has an unpaired electron and thus is highly reactive, as discussed in detail in Ch. 2.

Gamma Rays: Medium- to very high-energy, highly penetrating electromagnetic radiation emitted by radioactive materials. Can cause mutations, cancer, and birth defects.

Gray: The new measure of the dose of ionizing radiation *received* by living matter in terms of the energy deposited in a given amount of tissue; one gray equals 1 joule per kilogram of tissue. (One gray = 100 rads).

Half-life: The length of time required for half of the atoms of a radioactive element to decay to a different form. Note that this decay is exponential, not linear; after 2 half-lives, $1/4$ of the original element is left; after 3 half-lives, $1/8$; and after 10 half-lives, $1/1024$.

Ion: An atom or molecule which carries an electric charge: positive if it has lost one or more electrons, negative if it has gained one or more electrons.

Ionizing Radiation: Radiation whose energy is great enough to knock negatively charged electrons out of their atoms, thus disrupting atomic structures and leaving positively charged ions behind, causing a variety of kinds of damage in the process.

Isotopes: Different forms of an element which have the same number of *protons* but different numbers of *neutrons* in their nucleus. For example, radioactive carbon 14 differs from the much more common stable isotope carbon 12 in having 8 rather than 6 neutrons, while both have 6 protons (which is what makes them both carbon). Different isotopes of the same element have the same chemical and biological properties; only their physical properties are different.

Mutation: Damage to DNA, leading to a change in its sequence and thus loss or change either in a protein product or in some control step in producing that protein.

Neutrons: Neutral particles the same size as protons, which help make up the nuclei of cells. They also can be ejected at very high energy during the course of radioactive decay of some radioisotopes, are highly penetrating, and can cause genetic damage, cancer, and birth defects, as well as be used in radiation therapy.

Person-Rads: A measure of the collective dose of radiation received by a group of people. Thus, 100 person-rads may be one person receiving 100 rads of radiation, or 100 people receiving an average of one rad each.

Proton: The positively charged particles which are one of the two major components of the nucleus of each atom. The number of protons determines the kind of atom, and thus its chemical properties.

Proto-Oncogene: A gene in a normal cell which is identical with, or similar to, the cancer-causing genes (oncogenes) of tumor viruses. It is believed that carcinogenesis is the result of the alteration of structure or control properties of these proto-oncogenes.

Rad: Radiation absorbed dose, the older unit for measuring the dose of ionizing radiation in terms of the energy deposited in a given amount of tissue. (1 rad = 100 ergs of energy per gram of tissue.)

Radioactive Decay: The transformation of an atom of one element to an atom of another element through the release of ionizing radiation.

Radioisotope: A specific form of a given element which is unstable or radioactive and will thus tend to undergo radioactive decay to another element.

Rem: Different forms of ionizing radiation produce different amounts of damage to human tissue for the same total amount of energy, or rads. The unit rem takes this into consideration and describes the relative biological impact of the radiation being considered. It is approximately equal to the effect of one rad of gamma rays or 10 rems of more damaging alpha radiation.

Ribonucleic Acid (RNA): The linear polymers which are made in the nucleus of each cell as "Xerox copies" of the particular genes which that cell needs to use and which act as the direct templates for that cell's protein synthesis. The nucleotides of which RNA is made break down eventually to form uric acid, an antioxidant which, however, can produce gout when the levels are too high.

Roentgen: The earliest measure of the potency of ionizing radiation; it measures the amount of ionization induced in air. One roentgen is approximately equal to 0.88 rads.

Sievert: The new unit for measuring radiation dose while taking into consideration the relative biological impact of the radiation. One sievert is equal to 100 rems, and is approximately equal to one gray of gamma radiation.

Therapeutic Ratio: The ratio between damage to cancer cells and lethality of healthy tissue during radiation therapy (see Figure 7).

Tumor Promoter: Anything which can enhance the rate of growth of tumors; tumor promoters may or may not also be carcinogens.

X-rays: Man-made, highly penetrating, medium- to very high-energy ionizing electromagnetic radiation. Similar to gamma rays.

BIBLIOGRAPHY

General Books

American Cancer Society Massachusetts Division, 1982. *Cancer Manual,* 6th edition. B. Cady, M.D., editor-in-chief.

Committee on Diet, Nutrition and Cancer, U.S. National Academy of Sciences, 1982. *Diet, Nutrition and Cancer.* Washington, D.C., National Academy Press.

Poch, D., 1985. *Radiation Alert.* New York, Doubleday.

Prasad, K., editor, 1984. *Vitamins, Nutrition and Cancer.* New York, S. Karger.

Specific References

Agranoff, B., 1986. Inositol Trisphosphate and Related Metabolism. *Federation Proceedings* 45:2627–2628, 2629–2652.

Ames, B., 1983. Dietary Carcinogens and Anticarcinogens: Oxygen Radicals and Degenerative Diseases. *Science* 221:1256–1264.

Ames, B., R. Cathcart, E. Schwiers, and P. Hochstein, 1981. Uric Acid Provides an Antioxidant Defense in Humans Against Oxidant- and Radical-Caused Aging and Cancer: A Hypothesis. *Proceedings of the National Academy of Sciences of the United States of America* 78(11):6858–6862.

Badiello, R., 1970. Pulse Radiolysis of Selenium-containing Radioprotector. I. Selenourea. *International Journal of Radiation Biology* 17(1):1–14.

Barrie, S., J. Wright, J. Pizzorno, E. Kutter, and P. Barron, 1987. Comparative Absorption of Zinc Piccolinate, Zinc Citrate, and Zinc Gluconate in Humans. *Agents and Actions* (in press).

Basu, T., and C. Schorah, 1981. *Vitamin C in Health and Disease.* New York, Croom Helm.

Beckman, C., R. M. Roy, and A. Sproule, 1982. Modification of Radiation-Induced Sex-Linked Recessive Lethal Mutation Frequency by Tocopherol. *Mutation Research* 105:73–77.

Bland, J., 1982. *Choline, Lecithin, Inositol and Other "Accessory" Nutrients.* Volume 1. New Canaan, Connecticut, Keats.

Bland, J., 1984. Copper Salicylates and Complexes in Molecular Medicine. *International Clinical Nutrition Review* 4:130–134.

Bland, J., 1984. *Bioflavonoids.* New Canaan, Connecticut, Keats.

Booker, J., 1983. *Nutrition and Cancer.* BIS Thesis, University of Waterloo, Ontario, Canada.

Borek, C., A. Ong, H. Mason, L. Donahue, and J. Bigalow, 1986. Selenium and Vitamin E Inhibit Radiogenic and Chemically Induced Transformation *In Vitro* Via Different Mechanisms. *Proceedings of the National Academy of Sciences of the United States of America* 83:1490–1494.

Borish, E. T., and W. A. Pryor, 1987. Cigarette Smoking, Free Radicals, and Free Radical DNA Damage. *Annals of Internal Medicine* 107:526–545.

Bounous, G., 1983. The Use of Elemental Diets During Cancer Therapy. *Anticancer Research* 3:299–304.

Brekhman, I., 1980. *Man and Biologically Active Substances.* Elmsford, New York, Pergamon Press.

Burton, G., and K. Ingold, 1984. B-Carotene: An Unusual Type of Lipid Antioxidant. *Science* 224:569–573.

Cathcart, R., 1985. Vitamin C: The Nontoxic, Nonrate-Limited, Antioxidant Free Radical Scavenger. *Medical Hypotheses* 18:61–77.

Chaitow, L. 1985. *Amino Acids in Therapy.* New York, Thorsons.

Chaitow, L. 1985. *Could Yeast Be Your Problem?* London, Thorsons.

Cheraskin, E., and W. Ringsdorf, 1977. *Diet and Disease.* New Canaan, Connecticut, Keats.

Cheraskin, E., W. Ringsdorf, Jr., K. Hutchins, A. Setyaadmadja, and G. Wideman, 1968. Effect of Diet upon Radiation Response in Cervical Carcinoma of the Uterus: A Preliminary Report. *Acta Cytologica* 12(6):433–438.

Cheraskin, E., W. Ringsdorf, Jr., and E. Sisley, 1983. *The Vitamin C Connection: Getting Well and Staying Well with Vitamin C.* New York, Harper and Row.

Colombetti, G., 1969. *Studia Biophysica* 18(1):51–55.

Cook, G., and P. McNamara, 1980. Effect of Dietary Vitamin E on Dimethyl Hydrazine–Induced Colonic Tumors in Mice. *Cancer Research* 40:1329–1331.

Copeland, E., 1977. Intravenous Hyperalimentation as an Adjunct to Radiation Therapy. *Cancer* 39:609–616.

Copeland, E., 1979. Nutrition, Cancer, and Intravenous Hyperalimentation. *Cancer* 43:2108–2116.

Danetskaia, E., L. Lavrent'ev, N. Zapolskaia, and L. Teplykh, 1977. Kaltsiia fosfornokislogo po vykhodu opuholet pri odnokratnom: Khronicheskom deistvii smesi strontsii-90. *Voprosy Onkologii* 23:57–61.

Deretic, V., J. F. Gill, and A. M. Chakrabarty, 1987. Alginate Biosynthesis. *Biotechnology* 5:469–477.

Doege, T., and W. R. Hendee, 1987. A.M.A. Council on Scientific Affairs Report on Radon in Homes. *Journal of the American Medical Association* 258:668–672.

Edwards, M., 1987. Chernobyl—One Year After. *National Geographic* 171:633–653.

Fang, Y., Y. Lai, and W. Cao, 1983. The Effect of Vitamin B_{12} and Folic Acid on Radiation Damage. 3. Nitrogen Metabolism. *Acta Nutrimenta Sinica* 5(4):347–352.

Goodman, D., 1984. Vitamin A and Retinoids in Health and Disease. *New England Journal of Medicine* 310(16):1023–1031.

Greenwald, P., A. Ershow, W. Norelli, and C. Benton, editors, 1985. *Cancer, Diet, and Nutrition: A Comprehensive Sourcebook.* Chicago, Marquis Professional Publications.

Hernuss, P., E. Mullerty, H. Salzer, H. Sinzinge, L. Wicke, T. Prey, and L. Reising, 1975. Pollen Diet as an Adjuvant to Radiotherapy in Patients with Gynecological Carcinoma. *Strahlentherapie* 150(5): 500–506.

Hohenemser, C., M. Deicher, H. Hofsass, G. Lindner, E. Recknagel, and J. Budnick, 1986. Agricultural Impact of Chernobyl: A Warning. *Nature*, 321:817.

Hurley, L., and R. Shrader, 1975. Abnormal Development of Preimplantation Rat Eggs After Three Days of Maternal Dietary Zinc Deficiency. *Nature* 254:427–429.

Kahn, C., 1985. *Beyond the Helix: DNA and the Quest for Longevity.* New York, Times Books, Random House.

Levenson, S., C. Gruber, G. Rettura, D. Gruber, A. Demetriou, and E. Seifter, 1984. Supplemental Vitamin A Prevents the Acute Radiation-Induced Defect in Wound Healing. *Annals of Surgery* 200(4): 494–512.

Machlin, L. J., and A. Bendich, 1987. Free Radical Tissue Damage: Protective Role of Antioxidant Nutrients. *The Federation of American Societies for Experimental Biology Journal* 1:441–445.

Maisen, J., P. Dumont, and A. Dunjic, 1960. Yeast RNA and Its Nucleotides as Recovery Factors in Rats Receiving Whole-Body Radiation. *Nature* 186:487–488.

Marshall, E., 1987. Hanford's Radioactive Tumbleweed. *Science* 236: 1616–1620.

Marshall, E., 1987. Recalculating the Cost of Chernobyl. *Science* 236:658–659.

Maugh II, T., 1974. Vitamin A: Potential Protection from Carcinogens. *Science*, 186:1198.

Mester, A., 1983. Selective Modification of Glutathione Metabolism. *Science*, 220:474–477.

Meister, A., M. Anderson, and O. Hwang, 1986. Intracellular Cysteine and Glutathione Delivery Systems. *Journal of the American College of Nutrition* 5:137–151.

Ott, J., 1982. *Light, Radiation, and You.* Old Greenwich, Connecticut, Devin-Adair.

Park, E. Y., B. S. Luh, and A. L. Branen, 1984. Phenoloxidase and Antioxidant in Korean Ginseng. In: *Proceedings of the Fourth International Ginseng Symposium.* I. L. Heu, editor. Daejon-Shi, Korea, Korea Ginseng and Tobacco Research Institute.

Pauling, L., 1986. *How to Live Longer and Feel Better.* New York, Avon Books.

Pearson, D., and C. Shaw, 1983. *Life Extension.* New York, Nutri Books.

Peichev, P., 1966. Use of Apiary Products In Elderly Persons. *Folia Medica* (Bulgaria), 8(6):77–82.

Petkau, A., 1980. Radiation Carcinogenesis from a Membrane Perspective. *Acta Physiologica Scandinavica, Supplement* 492:81–90.

Pfeiffer, C., 1975. *Mental and Elementary Nutrients.* Keats.

Philpott, W., 1983. Oklahoma City, Oklahoma, Philpott Medical Center.

Pizzorno, J., and M. Murray, 1986. *Textbook of Natural Medicine.* Seattle, Washington, John Bastyr College Press. V:Vit A, 6.

Prasad, K., and B. Rama, 1983. Modification of the Effect of Pharmacological Agents on Tumor Cells in Culture by Vitamin C and Vitamin E. In: *Modulation and Mediation of Cancer by Vitamins.* F. Meyskens and K. Prasad, editors. New York, S. Karger, 244–257.

Prasad, K., and B. Rama, 1984. Modification of the Effect of Pharmacological Agents, Ionizing Radiation and Hyperthermia on Tumor Cells by Vitamin E. In: *Vitamins, Nutrition and Cancer.* K. Prasad, editor. New York, S. Karger, 76–104.

Prasad, K., P. Sinha, M. Ramanujam, and A. Sakamoto, 1979. Sodium Ascorbate Potentiates the Growth Inhibitory Effect of Certain Agents on Neuroblastoma Cells in Culture. *Proceedings of the National Academy of Sciences of the United States of America.* 76:829–832.

Pryor, W. A., 1970, 1973. Free Radicals in Biological Systems. *Scientific American*, August, 1970. In: *Organic Chemistry of Life*. M. Calvin, editor. New York, W. H. Freeman, 428–438.

Ringsdorf, W., and E. Cheraskin, 1980. The "Ideal" Daily Human Iodine Requirement. *Journal of Orthomolecular Psychiatry* 9:105–106.

Saksonov, P., 1975. Antiradiation Protection. In: *Foundations of Space Biology and Medicine*. O. Gazenko and M. Caldwin (eds.). Moscow, Nauka, 317–347.

Sarria, A., and K. Prasad, 1984. Tocopheryl Succinate Enhances the Effect of γ-Irradiation on Neuroblastoma Cells in Culture. *Proceedings of the Society for Experimental Biology and Medicine*, 175:88–92.

Scheef, W., 1979. *Cancer News Journal* 14(2):30.

Slater, T. F., K. H. Cheeseman, and K. Proudfoot, 1984. Free Radicals, Lipid Peroxidation and Cancer. In *Free Radicals in Molecular Biology, Aging and Disease*. D. Armstrong et al., editors. New York, Raven Press, 293–305.

Sorenson, J. 1986. Copper Combats Radiation. *The New Scientist* 110(1512):28.

Sternglass, E., 1986. The Implications of Chernobyl for Human Health. *International Journal of Biosocial Research* 8:7–36.

Sugahara, T., H. Nagata, and T. Tanaka, 1966. Effect of an Alkaline Hydrolised Product of Yeast on Survival of Repeated Irradiated Mice. *Radiation Research* 29:516–522.

Szorady, I., 1963. Pantothenic Acid: Experimental Results and Clinical Observations. *Acta Paediatrica* 4(1):73–85. Quoted in *Natural Healing*. M. Bricklin, editor. Emmaus, Pennsylvania, Rodale Press, 1976.

Takeda, A., M. Yonezawa, and N. Katoii, 1981. Restoration of Radiation Injury by Ginseng. I. Responses of X-Irradiated Mice to Ginseng Extract. *Journal of Radiation Research* 22:323–335.

Tappel, A. L., 1980. Vitamin E and Selenium Protection from in Vivo Lipid Peroxidation. In: *Micronutrient Interactions: Vitamins, Minerals and Hazardous Elements*. O. A. Levander and L. Cheng (eds.). *Annals of the N. Y. Academy of Sciences* 355:18–31.

Tato, L., M. Chiesa, and A. Zambone, 1987. Unexpected Lesson from Chernobyl. *Lancet* 1:803.

Tsao, C. S., 1984. Ascorbic Acid Administration and Urinary Oxalate. *Annals of Internal Medicine* 101:405–406.

Upton, A. C., 1982. The Biological Effects of Low-Level Ionizing Radiation. In: *Cancer Biology: Readings from Scientific American*. San Francisco, W. H. Freeman.

Wagner R., and E. Silverman, 1984. Chemical Protection against X-Radiation in the Guinea Pig. *International Journal of Radiation Biology* 12:101–112.

Webb, T., and T. Lang, 1987. *Food Irradiation: The Facts.* London, Thorson's.

Webb, T., T. Lang, and K. Tucker, 1987. *Food Irradiation: Who Needs It?* Rochester, Vermont, Thorsons.

Williams, R., 1979. *Biochemical Individuality.* Austin, Texas, University of Texas Press.

Wilson, R., 1987. A Visit to Chernobyl. *Science* 236:1636–1640.

Special Note

For a more detailed discussion of free radicals and their effects on biological systems, we refer you to the following technical publications:

Levine, S., and P. Kidd, 1985. *Antioxidant Adaptation.* San Leandro, California, Allergy Research Group.

Armstrong, D., R. Sohal, R. Cutler, and T. Slater, editors, 1984. Free Radicals in Molecular Biology, Aging, and Disease. *Aging* 27.

Cross, C., moderator, 1987. Oxygen Radicals and Human Disease (proceedings of the Davis Conference). *Annals of Internal Medicine* 107:526–545.

Lewis, D., and R. Del Maestro, 1980. An Approach to Free Radicals in Medicine and Biology. *Acta Physiologica Scandinavica, Supplement* 492:153–168.

INDEX

Accessory nutrients, 52–55, 93
Acetylcholine, 53–54
Acidophilus, 77
Adaptogens, 55–57, 93
Aging, premature, 1, 27
Algin, 72–74
Alpha-linoleic acid, 51–52
Alpha particles, 10, 15, 93
American Cancer Society, Massachusetts Division, 60
Amino acids, 43–46, 93
Antioxidants, 31–48
Antiradiation formula, Russian. *See* Russion antiradiation formula.
Arachidonic acid, 51
Ascorbic acid. *See* Vitamin C.
Atmospheric pollution, 20
Atomic number, 8, 9
Atomic structure, 6–8
Atomic weight, 10

Becquerel, Antoine Henri, 14
Becquerel (unit of measurement), 14, 93
Bedrock, radon gas in, 21, 81
Bee pollen, 57, 92
Bentonite, 75–76, 91
Beta-carotene, 32–34, 90, 91–92
Beta particles, 10–11, 93
Bile, 71
Bioflavonoids, 39–40, 90, 92
Biological units, 14
Birth defects, 1
Body, effects of free radicals, 19–29
  effects of radiation, 16–17, 60
  minimizing radiation damage, 49–57
Bones, cesium and strontium in, 71

Brain, 28, 53
Breast cancer, 37
Brewers' yeast, 39, 91
Building materials, radiation source, 80

Calcium, 75, 91
Calcium pantothenate, 38–39
Candida Albicans: Could Yeast Be Your Problem? (Chaitow), 39
Candida albicans infection, 39
Cancer, breast, 37
  skin, 5, 21
  nutrition in radiotherapy, 59–67
  radiation effects, 1, 21
  risk compared with radiation risk, 3
Cancer Manual, 60
Carbon 14, 69, 79
Carbon monoxide, 20
Carcinogenesis, radiation-induced, 26–27
Catalase, 40
Cells, 21, 24–26, 34
Cell growth, in cancer, 26–27, 60
Cell healing, 49–57
Cell membranes, interaction with free radicals, 23–24, 50
Cement, radiation source, 81
Ceramics, radiation source, 81
Cesium 137, 69, 71
Chaitow, Leon, 39, 43
Chemicals, source of free radicals, 20
Cheraskin, Professor Emanuel, 64–66
Chernobyl explosion, 1–2, 11, 28, 69–70, 74, 75
Choline, 53–55

Chromosome breakage, 24–26
Cigarettes, 2, 21, 81
Clay, 75–76, 91
Coal, carbon 14 in, 79
Color television sets, radiation
    source, 82–83
Copper, 40–41
Copper salicylate, 41
Cornell Medical Index, 74
Cosmic rays, 2
Counts per minute, 13
Curie, Marie, 13
Curie (unit of measurement), 13,
    94
Cysteine, 45, 92

d-alpha-tocopherol. See Vitamin E.
Decontamination, nuclear power
    plant, 2
Deoxyribonucleic acid. See DNA.
Dietary guidelines, radiation pro-
    tection, 90–92
Diet, Nutrition and Cancer, 3
Digestive system, role in removing
    radioactive substances,
    70–72
Disintegrations per minute, 13
DNA, radiation effects on, 1,
    16–17, 21, 24–26, 94
Dose fractionation, 60
Dosimeters, 86
Dry cleaning fumes, 20

EFAs, 50–52, 90, 94
Eicosapentaneoic acid, functions
    in body, 51–52
Electrons, 4, 6–8, 22, 94
Eleutherococcus, 56–57, 90
Encephalitis, atmospheric nuclear
    explosion effects, 28, 29
Energy, electromagnetic, 5
Environment, monitoring, 85–87
    radioactive material in, 69–77
Enzyme antioxidants, 40–43
Enzymes, 49–50
Essential fatty acids. See EFAs.
Europe, Chernobyl explosion ef-
    fects, 2, 28, 69–70, 75

Exhaust fumes, 20
Exponential notation, 94

Fertilizers, radiation source, 82
Film badges, 11–12
Fission chain reaction, 12
Flour, whole-grain, 21
Fluorescent lights, 84
France, after Chernobyl explosion,
    70
Free radicals, 94
    effects on cell membranes,
        23–24, 50
    effects on DNA, 24–26
    effects on proteins, 27
    effects on tissues, 19–29
    intracellular production, 21
    mechanism of damage, 22
    radiation-generated in vitamin C,
        63
    sources, 20–21
    structure, 7
Free radical deactivators, 31–48
Frequency, wave, 5

Gamma rays, 11, 94
Gamma-linoleic acid, 51
Geiger counters, 12–13, 85–86
Germany, after Chernobyl explo-
    sion, 70
Ginseng, 55–56, 90
Glass, optical, radiation source,
    82
Glutathione, 43–44, 64, 91, 92
Glutathione peroxidase, 41–43
Granite, radiation source, 81
Gray, 14, 94

Half-life, 10, 94
Heart, radiation effects, 28
Hemoglobin, 20–21
Hiroshima, 1
Histidine, 45–46

Immune system, 28, 50, 51
Infant mortality, nuclear explosion
    effects, 28
Influenza, nuclear explosion ef-
    fects, 28

Infrared radiation, 84
Inositol, 53–55
Intestinal lining, radiation effects, 27
Iodine, 74, 91
Iodine 131, 69, 71
Iodized salt, protection against iodine 131, 74
Ions, 94
Ionizing radiation. *See* Radiation, ionizing.
Isotopes, 8, 10, 94
Italy, after Chernobyl explosion, 74

Kelp, 72–74, 91
Korean Ginseng and Tobacco Institute, 55

Lead, radioactive, 2
Lecithin, phosphatidylcholine-enriched, 54–55
Light, ultraviolet, 4
  visible, 4, 85
Linoleic acid, 50–51
Liver, glutathione production, 44
Lungs, radiation effects, 27–28

Magnesium, 75, 91
Manganese, 40–41
Medical diagnostics, 2, 15, 16, 44, 60, 65–66
Microwave ovens, 83, 84, 86
Minerals, in radiation protection, 90–92
  in radiation response, 65–66
Molecules, 7
Mucous membranes, 33
Muscles, 53–54
Mutation, radiation-induced, 1, 24–26, 94
Myelin sheath, 46

Nagasaki, 1
National Academy of Sciences National Research Council, *Diet, Nutrition and Cancer,* 3
Nausea, vitamin B_6 in, 92

Nerves, 46, 53–54
Neutrons, 8, 10, 94
New York City, epidemic encephalitis in, 28, 29
Niacinamide. *See* Vitamin B_3.
Nuclear power plants, 2, 86
  Chernobyl, 1–2, 11, 28, 69–79, 74, 75
Nuclear reactors, 70, 79–80
Nuclear weapons, 1, 70
Nutrasweet, 43
Nutrients, accessory, 52–55, 93
  role in cell healing, 49–57
Nutrition, role in radiation response, 64–66
  role in radiotherapy, 59–67
Nutritional status, radiotherapy effects, 66–67

Oil, rancid, 21
Oncogenesis, 26
Optical glass, radiation source, 82
Oxidation, effects on tissues, 19–29

PABA, functions in body, 55
Paint fumes, 20
Pantothenic acid. *See* Vitamin B_5.
Para-aminobenzoic acid. *See* PABA.
Particles, in electromagnetic radiation, 4
Pectin, 72
Periodic table, 8, 9
Person-rads, 94
Pesticides, 20
Pollen, 57, 92
Pollution, atmospheric, 20
Polonium, radioactive, 2
Polyunsaturated fatty acids, 24
Potassium, 40, 69
Power stations, 16
Phenylalanine, 43
Phospho-gypsum, 80
Phosphate fertilizers, 82
Phosphatidylcholine, 54
Photons, 4–5
Pneumonia, nuclear explosion effects, 28

Proteins, 27, 65
Protons, 6–8, 95
Proto-oncogenes, 26, 95
Pyridoxine. *See* Vitamin B$_6$.

Quercitin, 40

Rad, 14, 94
Radiation, background, 79–87
    and carcinogenesis, 26–27
    and cell damage, 23–24
    effects on body, 16–17
    effects on DNA, 24–26
    and free radical damage, 22
    and genetic changes, 1
    infrared, 84
    ionizing, 4–6, 8, 10–11, 94
        background, 79–83
        in body, 69–77
        and free radicals, 19–20
        low-level, 2–3
        in radiation therapy, 59–67
    measurement, 11–13
    medical diagnostic. *See* Medical
        diagnostics.
    nonionizing, 4–6, 83–85
    nutrient protection from, 31–48
    types, 4–6
Radiation Alert (Poch), 80, 83
Radiation protection methods,
    summary, 89–92
Radiation response, 64–66
Radiation strength, measurement,
    13–15
Radiation therapy, 59–67, 91–92
Radiation threshold, 3
Radicals, free. *See* Free radicals.
Radioactive decay, 10, 94
Radioactive materials, environmen-
    tal, 69–77
    dietary protection against, 91
Radioactivity, background sources,
    79–87
    characteristics, 8, 10–11
Radioisotopes, 69–77, 94
Radiotherapy. *See* Radiation ther-
    apy.
Radio waves, 4, 84

Radon gas, in bedrock, 2, 81
Rain, radioactivity in, 70, 71
Rheumatoid arthritis, 45
Rem, 14, 94–95
Riboflavin. *See* Vitamin B$_2$.
Ribonucleic acid. *See* RNA.
RNA, 46–48, 91, 95
Roentgen, 14, 95
Royal jelly, 57
Russian antiradiation formula, 36,
    40, 45, 46
Rutin, 40

Scandinavia, after Chernobyl ex-
    plosion, 70
Scintillation counters, 13
Scurvy, in United States, 36
Selenium, 37, 42–43, 73, 90, 92
Sievert, 14, 95
Skin, radiation effects, 27
Skin cancer, 5
Smog, 20
Smoke detectors, radiation source,
    82
Sodium alginate, 73
Stars, cosmic rays from, 2
Stress, vitamin C for, 36
Strontium 90, 69, 71
Sulfur compounds, radiation pro-
    tection, 24
Sunlight, 2, 5, 21, 83
Superoxide, in radiation-induced
    damage, 22
Superoxide dismutase, 40–41, 50

Television sets, 82–83
Therapeutic ratio, 59, 60, 62, 95
Thiamine. *See* Vitamin B$_1$.
Thyroid gland, 71
Tissues, body, radiation effects,
    19–29, 60
    minimizing, 49–57
Tissue healing, vitamin A effects,
    33
Tobacco smoke, 2, 21, 81
Tryptophan, 46
Tumors. *See* Cancer.
Tumor promoter, 95

Index

107

Ukraine, after Chernobyl explosion, 2
Ultraviolet radiation, 20–21, 83
United States, average radiation
exposure, 15–16
iodized salt, 74
scurvy, 36
Uranium 235, 11
Uric acid, 46–48, 91

Visible light, 85
Vitamins, antioxidant properties,
32–40, 65, 90–92
Vitamin A, 32–34, 61–62, 91
Vitamin B$_1$, 38, 91
Vitamin B$_2$, 38, 91
Vitamin B$_3$, 38, 91
Vitamin B$_5$, 38–39, 90

Vitamin B$_6$, 39, 90, 92
Vitamin C, 34–37, 40, 63, 90,
91, 92
Vitamin E, 37–38, 62, 76–77,
90, 91

Warner, Dr. Glenn, 61
Watch dials, radium, 83
Waves, in electromagnetic radia-
tion, 4–6
White blood cells, radiation ef-
fects, 27
Whole-grain flour, 21

X-rays, 96. *See also* Medical diagnostics.

Zinc, 40–41, 49–50, 90, 92

<u>NOTES</u>

NOTES

NOTES

NOTES

NOTES

NOTES

<u>NOTES</u>

NOTES